The Sandwich Generation

Caught between Growing Children and Aging Parents

The Sandwich Generation

Caught between Growing Children and Aging Parents

H. Michael Zal, D.O., F.A.C.N.

PERSEUS PUBLISHING

Cambridge, Massachusetts

Library of Congress Cataloging-in-Publication Data

Zal, H. Michael.
    The sandwich generation caught between growing children and
aging parents / Michael Zal.
        p.   cm.
    Includes bibliographical references and index.
    ISBN 0-306-44124-1
    1. Middle age--Psychological aspects. 2. Middle aged persons-
-Family relationships. 3. Life cycle, Human. I. Title.
    [DNLM: 1. Adult--psychology. 2. Aged. 3. Anxiety Disorders-
-psychology. 4. Mental Disorders--in adolescence. 5. Middle Age-
-psychology. 6. Parent-Child Relations.   BF 724.6 Z22s]
RC451.4.M54Z35   1992
155.6'6--dc20
DNLM/DLC
for Library of Congress   92-1420
                                                              CIP

ISBN 0-7382-0581-8

10 9 8 7 6 5

© 1992 Perseus Publishing
Published by Perseus Publishing
A Member of the Perseus Books Group

An Insight Book

Printed in the United States of America

In memory of

FRANK ZAL, Esquire

(1910–1968)

whose light continues to shine on me

Acknowledgments

It has taken a year to write this book. What a year it has been. My first book, *Panic Disorder: The Great Pretender,* was published in April 1990. The positive feedback from family, friends, colleagues, patients, and others was tremendous and helped maintain the momentum I needed to keep writing.

I have a store of wonderful memories. The beautifully written complimentary letters. The phone calls from individuals all over the United States asking for information and thanking me for letting them know that they are not alone. The heart-warming applause following my lectures. Being interviewed on radio. The positive book reviews. The book signing. The article in *Psychiatric News,* summarizing my talk in Chicago at the AOA Writer's Conference on Men's Health. The pride shown by the American Osteopathic Association when I spoke at their 95th Annual Convention and Scientific Seminar in Las Vegas, Nevada. The letters of rejection from Donahue, Oprah, and Carson. Being included in the PennBook celebration in Philadelphia. Through it all, I wrote, and wrote, and wrote.

I am thankful to Norma Fox, Executive Editor of Insight Books, for her encouragement and continued confidence in my ability as a writer. I am thankful to the Plenum staff for their responsiveness to my many questions. Special thanks to Herman Makler, senior production editor, for a job well done.

I have been in the private practice of psychiatry since 1970.

I have been writing on mental health topics since my residency in psychiatry. This book draws on the breadth of my psychiatric practice as well as many of the subjects that I have written on in the past.

Many thanks to the following publishers for allowing me permission to reprint portions of my works first published in their journals and books:

Acme Newspapers, Inc., for "Teen Suicide: Don't Ignore the Signals of Warning," *Main Line Times, Sunday*, May 11, 1986, p. 25; "Out to Pasture: Retirement Can Be a Time of Confusion," *Main Line Times, Sunday*, August 31, 1986, p. 19; and "The Female Alcoholic: Different Problems but Same Addiction," *Main Line Times, Sunday*, September 21, 1986, p. 26.

The American Osteopathic Association for "Adolescence—A Period of Explosive Turbulence," *Health*, Vol. 13, No. 1, September, 1967, pp. 6–11; and "Can a Teen-Ager Be Depressed?" *Health*, Vol. 16, No. 2, October, 1970, pp. 7–11.

Cliggott Publishing for "Growing Older in the 80's," *Osteopathic Annals*, Vol. 11, No. 1, January, 1983, pp. 50–56; and "The Climacterium and Mid-Life Crisis," *Osteopathic Annals*, Vol. 12, No. 2, February, 1984, pp. 67–73.

Compendium Publishing Company, Inc. for "Understanding The Elderly," *Osteopathic Medical News (OMN)*, Vol. III, No. 3, March, 1986, pp. 1, 47–49; "Teen Suicide" *OMN*, Vol. 4, No. 6, June, 1987, pp. 15; "Substance Abuse," *OMN*, Vol. 4, No. 8, September, 1987, pp. 28; "Adjusting to Parenthood," *OMN*, Vol. 4, No. 10, November/December, 1987, p. 50; "Four Stages of Life, Part I," *OMN*, Vol. 5, No. 7, July/August, 1988, pp. 28; "Four Stages of Life, Part II," *OMN*, Vol. 5, No. 8, 9/88, pp. 21; and "Eating Disorders," *OMN*, Vol. 8, No. 5, May, 1991, p. 20.

MRA Publications, Inc. for "Recognition and Management of the Suicidal Adolescent," *Family Practice Recertification*, Vol. 12, No. 11, November, 1990, pp. 103–122.

W. B. Saunders Company for "Depression in the Elderly Patient," *Difficult Medical Management*, Robert B. Taylor, M.D. (Ed.) (Philadelphia, 1991), pp. 187–194.

I continue to be grateful to my patients for their respect and their trust. Even after more than twenty years in psychiatric practice, I still delight in working with their problems and seeing their progress. In some ways, it is the fabric of their lives, as well as my writing, that has produced this book. None are mentioned directly. All vignettes combine information and show much poetic license to make certain clinical points.

My thanks to my friend and colleague, Sheldon P. Wagman, D.O., Assistant Director of Adolescent Psychiatry at Friends Hospital, Philadelphia, Pennsylvania. His expertise helped me clarify some of the issues in the section "What to Do If Your Teen Needs Mental Health Treatment" in Chapter 4. Also thanks to my colleague and friend, Bala Cynwyd internist Bruce I. Blatt, M.D., as well as my wife, Alice J. Zal, D.O., for reviewing the section "Health Worries" in Chapter 9 for medical accuracy and for their suggestions for the section "The Health Exam in Middle Age."

This book is in part about family relationships. I want to acknowledge my immediate family, not only out of pride, but also because without them I could not do many of the things I do. My thanks to my mother, Evelyn D. Zal, for her caring, generosity, and words of wisdom. My wife, Alice, and my "big kids," Michelle and Fredrick, still define my life. Their accomplishments have continued since I wrote my last acknowledgments section, for *Panic Disorder*, in 1989. Alice entered medical school at the beginning of middle age. She has now completed residency training in General Practice. She deserves much credit. My daughter, Michelle, has been living independently, attending graduate school in Nursing Administration at Villanova University, and continues to work full time as a pediatric nurse. My son, Fred, our third generation at the University of Pennsylvania, has graduated as a Design of the Environment major. Could I ask for more?

This book is dedicated to my father, the late Frank Zal, Esquire, with love and respect. He died in 1968 while still in middle age. He would be pleased to know that family, friends, and colleagues still remember him with respect, praise, and affection. His light continues to shine on me and influence my life.

As for myself, I am deeply immersed in middle age and already focusing on new goals for the future.

H. MICHAEL ZAL

Bala Cynwyd, Pennsylvania

Contents

Introduction. Midlife: A Perspective   **1**

I. GENERATIONS

1. The Dilemma of Middle Age. Nora:
   A Representative Case History   **7**

2. The Parent–Child Bond   **15**

   Animal Bonding Studies   16
   Theories of Human Attachment   17
      Vignette: The Ferocious Bear   17
   Guidelines for Bonding Success   20
   Maternal Deprivation   21
   Fathers and Significant Others   22
   Infancy: From Birth to Age One   23
   Early Childhood: From Age One to Six   24
   Latency: From Age Six to Twelve   26

II. THE HIGH-TECH GENERATION

3. Adolescence: A Period of
   Explosive Turbulence   **31**
      Vignette: Beth   32

Physical Development   33
Psychological Changes   34
Separation from Parents   34
    Vignette: Brian   36
Search for Identity   36
Group Membership   38
Mentors and Other Role Models   38
The Generation Gap   39
Parent–Adolescent Relationships   40
Resolutions   42
Guidelines for Success   44

4. Troubled Teens   47
    Vignette: Mark   47
Adolescent Suicide   47
Risk Factors   48
Warning Signs   50
Teen Suicide Prevention   51
Masked Depression   54
Substance Abuse   56
Eating Disorders   59
    Vignette: Heather   59
Schizophrenia   61
    Vignette: Paula   61
What to Do If Your Teen Needs
    Mental Health Treatment   63

**5. Young Adulthood:
The Twentysomething Generation   67**
New Anxieties and New Responsibilities   68
College Bound: A Parent's View   69
A Place of Their Own:
    A Young Adult's Perspective   72
Life Choices and Other Developmental Tasks   73
A New Parental Appreciation   79

The Parent–Child Bond in Young Adulthood   *80*
Guidelines for Success   *82*

6. Anxiety and Other Emotional Roadblocks in Young Adulthood   *85*

Anxiety Disorders in Young Adulthood   *86*
Manic-Depressive Illness (Bipolar Disorder)   *91*
Entering the Adult Years   *93*
The Age Thirty Transition   *94*

III. THE SANDWICH GENERATION

7. The Challenge of Middle Age   *99*

Vignette: Rob   *99*
The Middle-Age Dilemma   *100*
Menopause: A Time of Change   *102*
The Male Climacteric: Middle-Age Crazy   *104*
Theories of Middle Age   *105*
Guidelines for Success   *110*

8. Crisis Points in Middle Age   *115*

Vignette: The Jolly Roger Syndrome   *115*
Stress in the Marketplace   *117*
Vignette: Barry   *119*
Marriage and Other Relationships   *120*
Vignette: Charlotte   *123*
Divorce Prevention   *124*
Adjusting to Postparenthood: The Empty
   Nest Syndrome and Other Problems   *128*
Middle-Age Stress   *130*
Guidelines for Success   *133*

9. The Middle-Aged Mind and Body   *135*

Shattered Dreams and Expectations   *135*

Midlife Depression   *136*
Substance Abuse and Other Crutches   *139*
    Vignette: Jenny   139
Sexual Issues   *140*
Health Worries   *142*
The Middle Age Health Exam   *148*
Guidelines for Success   *151*

10. Middle-Aged Children and Their Aging Parents   *155*

Standing Alone   *155*
Role Reversal   *156*
Resolving Old Issues   *158*
    Vignette: Barbara and Her Mother   159
Acceptance and Appreciation   *160*
    Vignette: Margie and Her Father   163
Achieving a New Relationship   *164*
Mom and Dad Are Getting Old:
  How About Me?   *166*
Facing Your Own Mortality   *166*
The Loss of a Parent   *167*
Guidelines for Success   *169*

IV. THE TRADITIONAL GENERATION

11. The Golden Years   *173*

    Vignette: George   174
Coping with a Retired Parent   *175*
Grandparenthood   *179*
Creativity in Late Life   *180*
To Live Again: Life after the Death of a Spouse   *182*
Sex after Sixty   *185*

12. The Last Mile   *189*

Vignette: Emma   *189*
Understanding the Elderly   *190*
Dementia   *191*
Vignette: Sallie   *193*
Depression in the Elderly   *194*
Vignette: Marion and Tom   *196*
A Place to Live   *196*
Legal and Ethical Dilemmas   *201*
The Caregiver Role   *203*
Avoiding Stress and Burnout   *205*
Guidelines for Caregiver Success   *207*
Death with Dignity   *209*

13. Middle-Aged Wisdom   *211*

Why Didn't Someone Tell Me?   *213*
Therapy: Is It Really the Answer?   *214*
Don't Be Afraid of the Dark   *217*
Generations: What Do They Want
    from Each Other?   *219*
Guidelines for Success   *223*

References   *227*

Index   *241*

About the Author   *251*

Introduction

Midlife

A Perspective

Caught in the middle. The Sandwich Generation. These might well be the phrases to best define midlife. The middle-aged man and woman are enmeshed in their own inner struggles. They have just lost the illusion that they can do everything in life and will live forever. They are coping with the biological and physical changes of aging. They may not always like their new selves. They have worked hard all of their lives. The family dog has died. They are looking forward to some time for themselves. Much to their dismay, however, they find themselves tightly sandwiched between the needs and problems of their adolescent and young adult children, as they push toward independence, and their aging parents as they slowly slide into a more dependent role. The middle aged are further stressed by trying to be available to their spouses and meet the demands of their jobs. As they grapple with the realities of midlife, they often wonder about the meaning of life.

" . . . For those with normal life expectancies the middle years constitute the longest span of our lives. Childhood and adolescence are but a preparation and old age a postscript. In a certain sense the middle years are life itself, or what living is all about."(1) Over 50 million Americans, one-fourth the population, are considered middle-aged. "They earn most of the money, pay the bills, and most of the taxes, and make many of the decisions. Thus, the power in government, politics, education, religion, science, business, industry, and communication is often wielded not by the young or the old, but by the middle-aged."(2) In the 1990s the ranks of the middle-aged are being swelled by the Baby Boom generation.

Human growth and development can continue to the very end of the life cycle. Being middle-aged is handled differently by people. Some grumble about the change but slowly master their various anxieties and conflicts and develop a new balance. Most try to build on what they have and grow more settled and content. For some it is a true crisis. One extreme is what I call the "Jolly Roger Syndrome," in which all is abandoned and the person starts from scratch with new relationships and new occupational goals.

The parent–child relationship, with all of its tortuous twists and turns through the life cycle, is usually the longest, and most intense, interaction a person will have with another human being. Dynamically convoluted, at times ambivalent and empassioned, it can be both confusing and conflictual, and also deeply satisfying. No relationship is as potent or complex.

Relationships with people you love can sometimes be difficult. Communications between generations is often problematic. Children of all ages struggle to express their needs, wants, and feelings. As parents and caregivers you will struggle with the same issues. You may worry that you are not doing enough. Just as gender is anatomical and there are many acceptable ways to be a man or a woman, there is no one right way to be a parent or a caregiver. You are not a bad person if you do not live up to all your expectations. As long as your love and caring shine through, it does not matter if your technique is not perfect.

There are no courses to take to learn how to be a successful parent or caregiver. Few tell us what we will encounter along the way. The idea for the focus of this book came from my wife. When I was mulling over proposal ideas, she mentioned that when our children were young, she often looked to books, such as Arnold Gesell's *The First Five Years of Life* and Benjamin Spock's *Raising Children in a Different Time*, to help understand what was going on and to cope with the different stages of our children's development. This made me realize that people might like a book to help them with their parent–child relationships in midlife. I tested out the idea on various friends, colleagues, and patients. Each time, smiles appeared and faces lit up. They all responded, "Boy, I could use a book like that!" Well, here it is. Although I certainly do not put myself in the same expert class with Gesell and Spock, I hope that you will find this book useful in understanding what is happening to your adolescent and young adult children, yourself in midlife, and your aging parents.

The book takes a biopsychosocial, dynamic, and holistic focus. Adolescence, middle age, and the geriatric years can all be arduous times in the life cycle. During middle age, all three age groups come on stage at the same time to interact in the game of life. I have tried to give you an overview of these three developmental stages so that you can understand what is happening to each of the generations. Particular emphasis is placed on the various mental health problems that can occur during each of these life stages. Vignettes are used to illustrate various points. Although there are no magic solutions, I have included several sections called "Guidelines for Success," which I hope will offer you some practical, logical, and sensible suggestions to help you cope with the problems and choices of midlife.

Being middle-aged is not always easy. It can be an extremely stressful time. "Middle age is a time for coming to terms with the limitations of one's self, of one's loved ones, and finally of reality."(1) Have faith in yourself and take care of yourself. Share your feelings. Ask for support when you need it. Remember that you cannot control other people. On the other hand, you are only responsible for 50 percent of an interpersonal interaction. Don't give up. Time heals and changes things. Each day is a new opportunity for success. Hang in there. You'll get through it. You'll probably look back and be able to say, "I'm a survivor."

It's not hopeless. People and their problems are not unique. We all have the same basic needs. The nuances and the timing may be different, but the name of the game is the same. I hope that this book will strike an emotional chord and be helpful to many as they struggle with the challenges of midlife. I hope that it will show you that you are not alone in your middle-age dilemma.

Part I

GENERATIONS

Chapter 1

The Dilemma of Middle Age

Nora:
A Representative Case History

Nora was 49. Something was wrong. It felt physical. She often had pressure in her chest and felt faint and short of breath. It felt emotional. She was often tense and moody. At times she thought that she would lose control and burst apart. She visited her family doctor. Except for moderate hypertension, the results of her physical exam were normal. All the lab test findings were within normal limits. Maybe it was menopause? A psychiatric opinion was sought. The clinical diagnosis was depression and anxiety. The real issue was the dilemma of middle age.

Nora's worries and complaints were not unique. As with many people in the sandwich generation she felt caught in the middle between generations, responsibilities, needs, and expectations. "I'm trying to sort out my obligations to my children, to my husband, to our aging parents, to my career, and to myself," she said. Nora felt stressed and driven by an intense emotional pressure which she did not fully understand.

"At this point in my life, I expected that I would be growing old gracefully and that everything would be O.K. I always assumed that as I got older I would get wiser, mellow, and have the answers to some questions. I thought that I would know what to expect and what others expected of me. I felt that I would be a calm and cool person. Instead, I feel terrible inside. I'm not who I should be. I'm not in control." Her turmoil and confusion were influencing her work and her relationship with her husband, Don. Let's look at some of the people in her life and some of the problems fueling her anxiety and discontent.

The Children: Jose was 19 and a college student living out of town. She called several times a week and dumped her problems concerning her boyfriend, school, and girlfriends on her parents. Nora worried for days only to find out when she called back that Jose had already forgotten the crisis and gone on to a new day and new issues.

Ben was 23, married, and had two beautiful twin daughters. He and his wife, Dianne, had lived with Nora and Don for 10 months after they married. They then moved to North Carolina. Ben was now unemployed and had gotten into a fight in a bar and been arrested. He and Dianne had separated three months ago, and Dianne and the babies were living with her mother. Nora worried about them all.

Henrietta, 25, planned to marry in October. Fiancé Bob was a carpenter and worked sporadically. They had a 14-week-old baby son, Matthew. Henrietta, Bob, and Matthew all lived with Nora and Don, while they saved to buy a house of their own. At a time when she expected her life to be her own, Nora was cooking and cleaning for five all over again. "The only comfort is that all my friends are going through the same thing. When I was young, you moved out and didn't go back. Things are different with the kids today."

The Parent: Nora was concerned about her mother, Ethel, who was 72 and lived many miles away. She had had a mild stroke last year. She had been recently hospitalized due to lack of appetite, fatigue, and insomnia. No new physical diagnosis was made. She was told to seek counseling for depression. Nora described her mother as a wise, productive, intelligent, and religious woman who allowed no disagreement. Nora's father also had had a history of depression and hypertension. He had been a heavy drinker. Since her husband died 10 years ago, Ethel had been self-sufficient and independent. When Nora visited her in the hospital, she could see a change. For the first time, Ethel looked frail and older. Uncharacteristically, she cried in her daughter's arms and shared her fear that she would have another stroke alone in her apartment and die. Nora realized that she too was aging. She began to think about her own health, her own future, and her own mortality.

Nora found it hard to be a caregiver at a distance. Her first instinct was to ask her mother to move to her home in Philadelphia. Somehow she knew that the offer would be rejected. She did talk to her brother and was very firm about what she felt her mother needed. She also called a local agency and was able to get someone to stay with her mother in the evenings several days a week.

The Spouse: Don had taken a new hobby. He was fixing up the house and adding a new porch. Nora complained that it had become an obsession. "He spends 85 percent of his spare time on the house. I want to go out dancing. By the time we're done with the house, I'll be too old to enjoy myself. I'm getting older. I want to do some of the things that I want to do." In quiet moments, she wondered if Don still found her attractive and worried about gaining weight. His business commitments were also very time consuming. In spite of her resentment, she worried about his health. He smoked one-and-a-half packs of cigarettes a day and had had a heart attack four years ago. She wondered what would happen if he had another health crisis and what life would be like without him. "It seems that he and I are always faced with something. We don't have time for each other."

The Inlaw: Don's father, Joseph, age 78, had been retired for many years. His wife, Camille, had died four years earlier after a long illness. Initially, Joe seemed to be making a good adjustment. Unlike many men his age, he had some hobbies and interests and played cards once a week. During the last year, his memory had been declining. Twice he had left the oven on overnight. His prostate had been removed, leaving him incontinent, and his vision was failing. Nora and Don constantly talked about the options that were available for Joe, including placement in a nursing home. They could never seem to make a decision.

The Job: Nora was well respected at the office. She had worked hard for many years and was now a manager supervising 12 employees. She was taken aback at times when they called her "Mame" and complained that the "kids" were not as diligent about their work as she and her contemporaries were at their age. There had been some recent administrative changes which added to the turmoil at work. There was talk of further changes and possible layoffs. Nora handled the pressure by working harder and taking on more responsibility. She felt tense, insecure, and irritable. When told that she had high blood pressure, she responded that she had no time to be sick.

Job security was important to Nora. She had heard many stories about her parents suffering during the Depression. The recent upheaval at work also created tension for her because it threatened a hidden agenda in her life. "When I took this job, I thought that I had finally reached a pinnacle in my career. I've been in a fast track mode. I thought that this might finally be the end of the line employment-wise. I could stay here. It would be a nice way to end my career and eventually retire. I wanted to stop work at 55. I would still have energy and still be young enough to enjoy the things we postponed all these years. They're messing up my life. If I have to start a new job at my age, it will shatter my plans." Even more confusing to her was the fact that she sometimes woke up at night and thought, "Maybe I'll give up my career and do some other kind of work."

As you can see, it is not surprising that Nora felt stressed and out of control. Her frustration was further fueled by her unfulfilled expectations. After early financial and marital struggles, the trials and tribulations of caring for children and attending to career goals, Nora, at 49, expected to be able to coast for awhile. Instead, she was caught between demanding children, a frightened parent, a needy father-in-law, and her own needs and desires. Her marriage was drifting. At this stage in life, she expected that she would feel mellow and content. Instead, she felt conflicted and needy. Instead of a rest, she had new problems to solve. No wonder she was angry inside.

More traditionally oriented, like her mother, it had been difficult for Nora to cope with a grandchild born out of wedlock and a son who was not particularly goal-directed. She joked and called him a "free spirit," but was really quite disappointed in him. Prior to therapy, Nora had assumed that at her age she was done learning and changing. However, life is synonymous with change. This too was part of her frustration. Change was difficult for her. Middle age is a developmental stage where we can resolve old issues and continue to mature and grow. She had to accept these truths. Nora found that even in middle age she had conflicts to resolve, new feelings to understand, and new problems to solve. She started to see middle age as a challenge. She did well.

Medication helped improve her mood and calm her anxieties. In therapy, she became a little more introspective and gained new insight through her reflections. She was able to ventilate some of her anger and understand some of her other feelings. She got her younger brother to spend more time with Ethel. She started to set some limits on Henrietta and Bob and asked for more help around the house. The "kids" moved to their own house in November. Nora expressed some of her pent-up anger and disappointment at Ben and told me how she felt that he had let her down. She tried hard to encourage Jose to solve some of her own problems and to be more independent. Most of all, she tried not to feel guilty if she could not be everything to everyone.

At work, she started to see herself in a new role as a consultant who had much experience and expertise to share but who no longer had to do it all herself. She started to delegate more.

Seventeen years earlier, she and Don had gone for marriage counseling. At the time, Nora had been depressed and unhappy. In a short course of outpatient therapy, she was able to come out of her depression and better communicate her needs. At this stage of her life, she again felt suddenly insecure and alone. She very much needed Don and felt resentful that he could not see this on his own and pay more attention to her instead of the house. Now, after 28 years of marriage, she could be more insightful. "It's happening again," she said. Fortunately, with a little therapeutic encouragement, she was able to talk to Don. She told him what she wanted from him and how much she cared. They started to take walks together and even went dancing one Saturday night. Their relationship started to improve again.

In therapy, Nora reminisced about her father's love of music. He had often sung and played the guitar for his children. She remembered how relaxing it had been in her childhood home when her father played operatic music on their Victrola. She bought a compact disc player and started to enjoy music again. As she relaxed, a more creative side emerged. She worked in the garden more and talked about taking a course in flower arranging. She started to see the big picture and put things in perspective. "I can't get so crazy. I have to take one day at a time. I'll do what I can for others and take better care of me." Although still uptight at times, Nora started to feel more content and more in control. She even took her antihypertensive medication regularly. Life was not perfect but it was much improved.

Nora is representative of many of you in the sandwich generation. The fabric of her life is made up of relationships. Her children and the other members of her family are important to her. She also has her own needs and priorities and wants to continue to grow. Her worries about her health and her future are universal. She has certain expectations about life in middle age. Her dilemma is not unique. In spite of the current turmoil and the angry feelings, a special bond of love exists between Nora and her family which will endure forever.

Before we look at the three most significant pieces of the middle age sandwich—you, your growing children, and your aging parents—let's take a look at the parent–child bond, which holds them all together.

Chapter 2

The Parent–Child Bond

The child, from the moment of birth, is irrevocably bound to its parents biologically and emotionally. Physical separation by geographical distance, personal choice, or even the death of a parent does not change this bond. Much of the joy and sorrow of life revolves around this attachment and the strong emotional states it engenders. The parent–child interaction is a dynamic drama that continues over the lifespan, enriching the process of human development. The nuances of the relationship may change as each person grows and matures over time. However, children and parents remain intimate and interdependent. In all stages of life, they continue to influence each other through this emotional investment.

As we saw in Chapter 1, Nora and her family members, three generations at three completely different points in their lives, still are greatly influenced by these strong affectional ties, rich in feelings of love, concern, and devotion. The term "attachment" was coined by John Bowlby, an English psychoanalyst, in 1958 to define this emotional tie that one family member has for another. A selective attachment that is established during the first six months of life is called *bonding*. This unique relationship between two people persists over time, even during periods of absence. It gives a child a feeling of basic security. Initially, it provides a source of strength and identity. Later, it serves as a point of detachment or separation. It is a paradox of development that the most securely attached child finds it easiest to separate and become independent. A satisfactory attachment of the child to the caregiver is the cornerstone of all future development.(1)

Animal Bonding Studies

Animal research models have been used to explore this connection. Konrad Lorenz is known for his studies of imprinting in animals. *Imprinting* is a social attachment in animals that develops quickly during an early "critical or sensitive period" following birth. Lorenz described how newly hatched goslings are programmed to follow a moving object (usually the mother). This form of learning often influences behavior in later life and is particularly resistant to change.(2) Although there is no evidence that supports the phenomenon of imprinting in humans, we do know that once a child has learned to trust and attach to one person, it is easier to bond to a second person.(1)

Psychologist Harry Harlow brought the science of primatology into the world of clinical psychiatry. His studies of attachment and separation between infant rhesus monkeys and cloth or wire-covered surrogate mothers showed that they were physiologically equivalent but not psychologically equivalent. Contrary to what we may expect, the baby monkeys preferred the cloth mother over the wire mother who fed them. "Contact comfort" was more important than feeding in bonding these infants to their surrogates.(2,3) Harlow's work shattered the earlier "need theory," which postulated that the provision of food and attention to physiological need satiation was the basis of attachment. Harry and Margaret Harlow proved that there is more to attachment than just being fed adequately. Providing comfort is a much stronger and more important force in stimulating significant human relationships.

Theories of Human Attachment

Attachment behavior, or the process by which a child establishes a close relationship with its parents, has been studied by many. Sigmund Freud(4) used the concept of object relationships to explain human attachments. He felt that the infant, a self-centered organism, develops an awareness of some external object whom it feels can fulfill instinctual needs and reduce tension. The infant invests its libidinal and aggressive energies into this object, usually the mother. Positive feelings come to be associated with this person, who becomes the child's first love object. This relationship becomes the prototype of all future love or object relationships. If the baby's needs are satisfied, he or she learns to love. Later the child can love and be loved. If he or she is frustrated, this feeling can also be transferred to other relationships. Borderline personality disorders and psychotic individuals, whose egos have been distorted or arrested in development, evidence a stunted and immature capacity for object relationships.

Vignette: The Ferocious Bear

During my residency training in psychiatry, I treated a 28-year-old single man who had great trouble dealing with the therapeutic relationship. He caused me much anxiety. He also taught me a lot about the parent–child bond and relationships. John Lenard was a large man six feet four inches tall and weighing over 225 pounds. He came to therapy reluctantly. He often skipped sessions and would show up the next week, unexpected, at his regular time. When he did come, he spent the session impressing me with his knowledge of engineering and electronics, of which I knew very little. On the surface, he appeared bright; however, he had very little substance or empathy for others. He looked like the male equivalent of a bag lady.

It was difficult to get John to talk about himself or his life. Over time, I learned that he lived with his father, who paid very little attention to him. His mother was deceased. He had no friends and had never been employed. He spent his time in a room cluttered with magazines and newspapers. The radio was often the only voice he heard. At other times, he wandered aimlessly through the streets, not speaking to anyone.

When particularly stressed in therapy, John would get up from his seat and move quickly around the room brandishing an umbrella at me. Frightened and intimidated, I tried to appear calm as I held on tightly to the sides of my chair. My supervisor nicknamed John "the ferocious bear." I gradually learned that his outrageous behavior covered up feelings of insecurity and inadequacy.

Although intelligent, John could not use his knowledge to build a meaningful life. One of his main deficits was his inability to make connections with others. He eventually shared some information that was important in understanding how he got to be the man I knew. John's mother had become very depressed right after his birth (I suspect a manic-depressive illness). She left John in the care of his nonnurturing father and went to recuperate for almost a year with her family in Chicago. No emotional bond was created between John and his parents. Without this, he had been stunted in his emotional growth and social development.

I never really felt that I had solved much for John in therapy. Many years later, I realized that perhaps I had given him more than I had originally thought. My time and attention had for a short time satisfied some of his existential loneliness.

Another approach to attachment behavior was taken by Erik Erikson, who proposed an eight-stage theory of psychosocial development.(5) Erikson felt that at each stage a conflict related to social relationships must be resolved. The first or infant stage, which is relevant to our discussion here, he called "trust versus mistrust." The infant's sense of trust is developed as the caregiver repeatedly satisfies needs for food, comfort, warmth, and touch. If the child learns that care and love are available in his world, he will maintain a hopeful attitude and can later generalize this social trust to others.

Another theory of development was suggested by researchers John Bowlby(6), a child psychiatrist, and Mary Ainsworth(7), an American psychologist. This theory blends psychoanalytic and ethological (the biological study of behavior) concepts. They believed that certain types of stimulation from the caretaker elicit certain behaviors in the infant. Conversely, certain infant behaviors elicit certain behaviors in the caretaker. Like Harlow, they felt that feeding plays a minor role in the development of attachment. Rather, they considered that reciprocal sensitive social feedback between infant and caretaker was a more critical component.

Bowlby described four phases in the development of attachment. The "preattachment" stage occurs during the first few weeks of life. During this time, the infant uses innate behaviors, such as rooting, sucking, grasping, crying, and following with the eyes to signal its needs and attempts to come in contact with the caregiver. The survival value of these behaviors facilitates the development of attachment. The second stage (3 to 6 months) is "attachment in the making." This begins when the infant can discriminate the primary caregiver from others. The child will respond differently to various people. Actions such as smiling and grasping are directed, coordinated reaching emerges, and family members will differ in their ability to get the baby to stop crying.

The third phase, "clear-cut attachment," occurs between 6 and 12 months of age. In this phase, the child can clearly discriminate between mother and others. He is more goal-oriented and actively seeks contact with the caregiver by locomotion. After his first birthday, the child starts to understand that mother is an independent individual whose behavior can be predicted. His view of the world thus becomes more realistic. Gradually, a more complex relationship develops between mother and child in which they start to influence each other's behavior. After 24 months of age, he enters the fourth phase by "formation of a goal-directed partnership" with the caregiver.

The parent–child bond may be instinctual or learned. However, "regardless of the theoretical interpretation used, . . . infants do form specific and primary relationships with adult caretakers, usually a parent and more specifically the mother. It also appears that infants and parents are mutually involved in the formation of the relationship."(8) Love is the ray of light that connects parent and child and warms them both. In a way, the work described above from Lorenz and Harlow to Freud, Erikson, Ainsworth, and Bowlby are really scientific studies on the topic of love. Successful early attachment will determine if the child will develop normally and feel secure. It is a symphony between parent and child that resonates trust and affection. Although the members of the system usually individuate by the time the child is three years old, if bonding is successful, they will continue to maintain heavy emotional ties to each other throughout life.

Guidelines for Bonding Success

The quality of parent–infant interaction appears to be profoundly influenced by early contact. Klaus and Kennell(9) postulated a biologically determined "sensitive period" for attachment and bonding in humans during the first few days following birth. There are certain mutually rewarding tools which facilitate parent–infant interaction and bonding.(1) Some of these may be innate and instinctual:

1. Talk to your infant. Babies appear to prefer a soft high-pitched voice.
2. Rock the baby.
3. Look at your infant. Full-faced eye-to-eye visual engulfing is best ("attending behavior").
4. Smile at the baby.
5. Hold your infant close and caress with a gentle relaxed touch ("enfolding").
6. As best you can, respond to and try to satisfy your baby's needs.

Maternal Deprivation

If the early attachment is not satisfactory or lacking, emotional problems can arise. The effects of maternal deprivation are particularly severe if they occur for long periods of time during the first two years of life. Rene Spitz studied this phenomenon. If there is loss of the mother during the second six months of life and no substitute caretaker is provided, the infant can develop an anaclitic depression.(10) The syndrome shows itself through weepiness, apprehension, withdrawal, refusal to eat, and sleep disturbances. It can even result in marasmus, stupor, and death. The term "anaclitic" refers to the "leaning-on" quality of the infant's relationship to the mother, who nourishes and cares for him. Spitz considered this condition the infant version of a depressive psychosis. If a caregiver is made available within three months, the child usually recovers.

Spitz(11) also studied institutionalized infants and found some to be apathetic, withdrawn, and severely depressed. They had elevated death rates, retarded physical and social development, and were emotionally immature. He referred to these symptoms of maternal and social deprivation as "hospitalism." Spitz's work stimulated the change from orphanage to foster home care in the United States.

Deprivation at this level can result in psychopathology characterized by a relative inability to maintain the love relationship in the face of frustration and to accept the limitations and separateness of the loved object. The capacity to love is a function that assumes increasing importance during normal maturation and development. An immature capacity for object relationship is characteristic of borderline personality disorders and psychotic individuals. In clinical practice, one sees a great many more cases of compromise, somewhere along the continuum of emotional development, than these pathological extremes. Some of these individuals will have difficulty dealing with people and often show problems expressing feelings such as love and anger.

If the love bond does not develop, the child can have trouble later in life making human connections. Intimacy, commitment, and caring may be difficult for him. Maternal separation or lack of social stimulation, as we saw in John Lenard's case, can interfere with the ability to form ongoing relationships. "Mature love . . . is characterized by a strong communicative relationship of openness, is high in caring and intimacy, and typically endures"(12).

Fathers and Significant Others

Until recently, fathers were seen as economic providers and involved themselves very little in the responsibility of child rearing. Many felt awkward even holding their infant. These attitudes and behaviors are changing as fathers take a more active role in nurturing activities. Even single-parent families headed by males are increasing. Previously, it was felt that only women, having been given a womb and breasts, could be a caretaker. As was shown in the Harlow monkey experiments, mothering not only involves nurturing in the sense of giving food but also includes the important component of comforting physical contact. If mothering is learned and refers to not only nurture in the sense of giving food but also to a total sense of training, educating, and rearing, then fathers could also assume such a caretaker role.(8)

In recent times, many fathers have become free to pursue this caretaker role. They seem to be interested in this new definition of fatherhood and enjoy the interaction. They involve themselves with physical caretaking tasks as well as the emotional involvement needed to establish a bond or affectional tie. Men are readjusting their images and becoming more secure in the knowledge that "the capacity to enrich and to actualize one's life through the experiences of another is not the prerogative of women. Feelings of tenderness and gentleness, the capacity to empathize and to respond emotionally to others, and the ability to value a love object more than the self are human characteristics."(13)

Most family members will rapidly develop strong unconditional positive warm feelings toward a new child in the home. Significant others involved in the child's upbringing, such as grandparents, older siblings, aunts and uncles, and even neighbors, can also play an important role in the child's development. In the initial phase of psychotherapy with adults, it is common for the therapist to ask the patient to describe some of the important people in his or her life. The therapist wants to see how the patient views them (not necessarily how they really are) and thus gets some idea of the patient's object relationships. At times a rather bland recitation is obtained in reference to Mom and Dad. It is only later when describing a grandmother or favorite aunt involved in parenting that a light goes on and the therapist can see where the love bond was established.

Infancy—From Birth to Age One

The early love bond or emotional attachment between human infant and primary caregivers, usually both parents, is a major event in the course of the infant's social development. During the first months and years of life, a flow of concern and affection is transmitted between parent and child which creates an affectional bond that may be the strongest of all human ties. The bond between the human baby and its parents develops during a critical period of time after birth in the same way that imprinting occurs in baby geese. "Contact comfort" is important for bonding in humans as well. During the first year of life, the infant is helpless and dependent. A symbiotic relationship unites the caregiver and the infant. Initially, the relationship is so intimate that the two seem to be almost one.

The power of this attachment is so great that it enables the mother and father to make the unusual sacrifices necessary for the care of their infant day after day.... This original parent–infant tie is the major source for all the infant's subsequent attachments and is the formative relationship in the course of which the child develops a sense of himself. Throughout his lifetime the strength and character of this attachment will influence the quality of all future ties to other individuals.(14)

The parent who protects the infant and fulfills its early needs helps build a feeling of basic trust and general security. The presence of a parent or other caregiver can serve to keep the child calm in a fearful or strange situation.

The emotional bond between parent and child developed during this period will lay the basis for all later personality development and continue to engender strong feelings through the years to come. "The unchallenged maintenance of a bond is experienced as a source of security and a renewal of a bond as a source of joy . . . the threat of a loss arouses anxiety and actual loss causes sorrow, while both situations are likely to arouse anger."(15) Separation from loved ones remains difficult for most people throughout their adult lives.

Early Childhood—From Age One to Six

The parent–child relationship is a constantly changing process. During infancy, the parent is primarily a nurturing, loving caregiver. By the end of the first year, the symbiotic mother–child unit is dissolved as the infant becomes a separate person and starts to strive for independence. Preschoolers start to develop autonomy but still depend on their parents to fulfill most fundamental physical and psychological needs. They will continue to require much love and attention. During childhood, however, the parent will also have to concentrate on teaching the child to act in ways that society considers acceptable. This process by which the child internalizes its parent's sense of right and wrong and society's attitudes, values, and customs is called *socialization*. It has a profound effect on social and personality development.(16)

This stage of development is characterized by self-assertion. The child learns to stand, walk, and run alone. Parents must encourage their independence but protect them against injury. Parental concerns now must involve safety and supervision. There is a growing ability to use and understand speech and acquire knowledge. Parents' active interest in cognitive and language development can greatly influence the child. The mastering of sphincter control occupies a special place in this phase of development. As the child shows an interest in bowel control and bowel products, a new drama develops between parent and child. The child quickly learns that he can please or easily frustrate the parent by his compliance or noncompliance. In some homes, this area can become a tense war zone. The preschooler also becomes involved in peer relationships individually and in groups. He starts to learn social skills such as cooperation, altruism, and the control of aggression. Parents should provide opportunities for him to make friends and provide the necessary playthings.

During ages one to six, the child also starts to develop an identification and a gender role. Initially, both girls and boys imitate the mother. Before long, the boy will turn toward a male identification figure such as his father, grandfather, or brother. Biology affects behavior and gender roles through the action of male and female hormones. We also learn male and female roles in part by imitating our parents or other adult models. The parents' gender expectations determine how they treat their child and subsequently also influence sex-role development.

According to classical psychoanalytical theory, during the third or fourth year of life, the child falls deeply in love with the parent of the opposite sex, develops intense jealousy toward his other parent, whom he sees as a competitor, and enters the oedipal phase of psychosocial development. The child develops the "grand illusion" of one day marrying a parent and having his or her child. This fantasy, the normal climax of a small child's identification with a like-sexed parent and his or her love for the other parent, is doomed to rejection, disappointment, and disillusionment. Anger is the natural response to frustration. The oedipal child must master anger and fears in relation to both parents, realign sexual and aggressive drives, and form more realistic fantasies. The child who is successful in resolving its oedipal conflicts will enter the next phase of development free from the overdependence of infancy and free from the frightening fantasies of parent retaliation for its forbidden loves and hates. He or she will be on his way to success in dealing with normal adult aggression and achieving normal adult love.(14)

Latency—From Age Six to Twelve

Somehow, the emotionally stormy oedipal period is resolved. The child enters the calmer period of latency and continues to focus on mastering the environment and herself or himself by entering school. Sexual preoccupation and unchanneled aggression become sublimated into general curiosity and learning.

> ... The phase of latency has within it inevitable sources of stress ... [which] arise from the daily separation from the family, from the necessity for adapting to the peer culture and the school system, and from the increasing demands made upon the child ... that he master new skills, exert more and more emotional control, acquire more and more knowledge, and enter into a number of new and often conflicting social roles.(17)

The parental bond will continue to give support and offer refuge when the outside world becomes frustrating. Parents will also help the child solve problems and make choices. Parental attitudes concerning achievement will have an impact on the child. Latency is a time of limits. Corporal punishment and child abuse of any kind should not be condoned. Parents, as well as religious instruction, if present, can play a critical role in setting limits. Discipline style as well as attitudes toward the expression of feelings (both hostility and affection) and toward sexual curiosity and experimentation will affect the child's values and self-esteem.

The bond between parent and child continues throughout the life cycle. Strong feelings prevail. Sometimes the effects are more subtle. At times the clash is heard loudly. Initially the infant is dependent on the adult. This balance gradually changes until, later in life, the adult becomes the caregiver for the parent. The parent–child relationship is the strongest and most involved tie of all, impinging on all phases of life.

This chapter has given an overview of individual psychosocial dynamics and interactive patterns between parents and children from infancy through latency. We hope that this would serve as an introduction. It may bring back many memories of your early interaction with your own children. You may wish to use it as a reference when you have grandchildren. We will continue to elaborate on the parent–child bond in the chapters to follow, as we explore some of the other major stages of life—adolescence, young adulthood, middle age, and old age.

Part II

THE HIGH-TECH GENERATION

Chapter 3

Adolescence

A Period of Explosive Turbulence

Nothing prepares you to be the parent of a teenager. You are never really ready for the tremendous changes involved. You watch with fascination as your offspring pass through infancy, childhood, and latency. You look on with pride as the baby lifts its head for the first time, the small boy enters school, and the young lady attends a birthday party dressed in organdy and lace. Each step is an achievement. Each achievement gives joy and serves as one of the rewards of parenthood. In typical parental fashion, the child's shortcomings and inadequacies are overlooked or minimized. All disappointments and difficulties are repressed and are soon overshadowed by the sweet promise of the future.

They are such lovely children. She is Daddy's little girl and Mommy's joy. He is the embodiment of every positive expectation. Before long, puberty bursts on to the scene. Hormones start to pump and it all changes abruptly as a period of explosive turbulence begins. Adolescence brings sweeping changes in outward physical appearance, emotional response, and behavior. At approximately age 12, a youngster enters a transitional period that will last a decade. New experiences produce new learning and improved social skills. The interplay of anatomical, physiological, emotional, intellectual, and social factors can create disequilibrium.

This metamorphosis affects both parent and child. Frustration is often the name of the game for the parent of a teenager. During this phase of development, the parent–child relationship undergoes many dramatic changes as the adolescent deals with the issues of identity, independence, and vocational choice. These changes alter your relationship forever and strain your bond. A struggle ensues between you that challenges all of life's customs and basic principles. Family life is pitted against group rituals and ideology. Parental praise changes to outrage and often outright condemnation as teenage ideals clash with adult convictions and expectations. One generation battles the other in a war of independence with a resultant change in equilibrium and at times a breakdown in family relationships.

Adolescence is one of life's most trying times for both parents and teenagers. Both must deal with awesome issues that do not always have perfect solutions. The friction between you can make matters ever worse. What is happening during this period of time? Why is it so difficult for all concerned? What is it that makes children rebel and appear to hate so much about their parents? What makes a loving and concerned parent suddenly dislike his or her child and draw back in indignation, disapproval, and anger? Both parent and child are fighting to transform the teenager into a mature adult who will have a satisfying, worthwhile, and meaningful life. Why is it that, with this common goal, parents and their teenage offspring seem to be pulling in two different directions? Could there be more than one road to maturity? The following vignette will help introduce some of the physical and emotional stressors that make up the adolescent experience.

Vignette: Beth

Beth was beautiful. She radiated a fragile innocence. She was like a flower newly in bloom. Adults stared at her in awe, but she felt that she was fat and ugly! At age 15, she was tall and unsure of her newly developed body. To make matters worse, her girlfriends were short and petite. Beth worried a great deal—about boys, about her school grades, about being accepted by her peers. At home, she was moody and demanding. She wanted to be a grown woman but was hesitant to take on new responsibilities, often wanting her mother to do it for her. Being 15 wasn't easy for Beth. Everything was a lot of pressure.

Physical Development

Adolescence is a time of physical growth and maturation. It is a time of accelerated changes in anatomic and physiologic capacity. Various biologic systems begin to function and influence the total organism. Previously dormant endocrine glands start to produce hormones that cause specific changes in growth patterns and physical appearance. Secondary sex characteristics, such as genital development, change in hair distribution, and voice changes, become apparent, and the child becomes an adult physically.

In both males and females, the order of these events as well as their time of onset vary widely. These alterations in appearance and physiology often prove confusing and frightening to the individual involved. Both the slowly maturing child and the precocious one may develop an anxious preoccupation as to the meaning or adequacy of these changes and their relationship to adult roles in society.

An empathic and understanding adult can be of great help to the adolescent in interpreting these changes in a friendly and casual way. Puberty can be traumatic. Bodies often grow in ways that are frustrating and confusing. If they are running late, they will need reassurance that their growth and development will catch up. If they are early, they may be embarrassed with underdeveloped peers, feel awkward, and wonder what is going wrong. Both may need reassurance that physical changes are following normal and expected pathways. Parents will have to reach back and remember their own feelings during this stage of growth to be able to be fully empathic.

Answer your child's questions about sex and physical development. This is hard for some. Many fathers, for instance, suggest "You'll have to ask Mom." Don't shuttle the child back and forth and cause him to exclaim, "I'm the kid in the middle. I'm all confused." Try to give a simple and direct answer to questions. The youngster will ask for more if he is not satisfied. Don't be afraid to voice your views and opinions. You and your child do not always have to agree.

Psychological Changes

Growing up, however, is more than just physical growth and development. Psychologically, the biophysiologic changes of puberty bring with them a quantitative increase in sexual and aggressive strivings as they reawaken the instinctual conflicts of infancy and early childhood. This causes a period of trial and error, during which the developing and maturing person is faced with numerous stresses. The teenager must deal with both internal and external input that do not always coincide. Conflicts abound in reference to instinctual strivings, self-concept, and moral teachings.

Separation from Parents

One of the main tasks an adolescent has is to separate from his parents and find his own identity. Detaching from parents is a necessary but often painful step toward maturity. Freud(1) described detachment from parental authority as the most significant and most painful psychic achievement of adolescence. Depression and loneliness can be a natural consequence of this psychic loss. Although wanting liberation, the teenager may at times feel that the parents have abandoned him. Ambivalence prevails. To reach his goal, he must finally relinquish the past and its former childhood pleasures.

Although verbally and behaviorally he seems to be screaming, "Mom and Dad, won't you let me go?", he longs for parental love and support. A strong internal instinct does not allow him to accept your help. Parents must try to respond to this inconsistent message. Tell him you are there if he needs you but let him take responsibility for his own actions. Your main task, as a parent, during this period is to let go. Your son or daughter will find his or her way and grow up in spite of your worries. The best thing you can do is set an example. Children tend to copy what they see and not what they are told.

Psychoanalytic theory explains what is happening in the parent–child relationship during this time as follows. Parents are the child's first love objects. With the advent of adolescence, they can no longer fulfill this role, unless an incestuous relationship develops. Anna Freud(2) commented that emotions play an important role in the struggle of the adolescent as he disengages himself from his parents and embarks on a search for new love objects. Most of the strong feelings he has for his parents have to be denied, and he experiences a sense of loss and loneliness. Feelings of both love and anger are turned toward the self. Adolescents become more narcissistic or self-centered, spending a great deal of time on themselves. Aggression or negative feelings can be externalized in behavior problems or contribute to feelings of depression or despair.

Initially, adolescents are still dependent on their parents for security, guidance, and financial and emotional support. As teenagers strive for independence, acquire new skills, and increase in physical size, the balance shifts and they increase their ability to exert power and control over parents. As parents discover their children becoming older and more self-sufficient, they are also undergoing their own physical and emotional changes. As is characteristic in transitional periods, the teenager may feel impatient, frustrated, intolerant, disorganized, and confused as he adapts and restructures behavior to accommodate a new direction in life course.

Tempers can flair as a new equilibrium evolves. The friction between parent and child can often cause profound anxiety and stress. Both parents and teenager will require understanding and support. Often, parents must learn to back off, at times without comment. Some rebellion is needed for growth and development. Since the adolescent stands midway between personal independence and continuing dependence on parents, many emancipatory acts occur. He may experiment periodically with various modes of self-expression which can frighten and concern the "grown-ups." In many areas, the adolescent will take pride in the differences between the two generations. Hopefully, when the dust settles, a new and mutual respect will have developed between mature adults.

Vignette: Brian

There he is, Mr. Teenage America. After an hour in the bathroom, Brian looked very together in his adolescent costume. His hair was combed. On his wrist were the mandatory friendship bracelets. Today he wore new jeans with pretorn holes in the legs and knees. A colorful cloth patched a hole over his buttock. The ensemble was completed by a surf teeshirt, high tops, and a "do rag" placed on his head. Tomorrow it could be army fatigues and combat boots. The next day might bring his leather jacket with all the zippers and a hanging earring in his left ear. He could not decide who he was or who he wanted to be.

Behind his cool facade, this tenth-grader was bristling with emotions. The critic inside shouted, "You don't look quite right today. Everyone will notice." Like most teenagers, he lived in the here and now. There was no tomorrow, only the immediacy of today. The possibility of dying of embarrassment was a daily event. Public humiliation could occur on the school bus, in the classroom, at a sporting event, and in every encounter with the opposite sex. Murphy's law plays a strong role in a teen's life.

Search for Identity

Brian is not unique. Growing adolescents, both male and female, are often preoccupied with how others see them and how they perceive themselves. This is basically a search for personal identity, a sense of self. If this is achieved, adolescents are able to plan a realistic future, with goals in education and vocation toward which they can effectively work.

Erik Erikson(3), a psychoanalyst and pupil of Anna Freud, worked with the concept of identity. He felt that "developmental change in adolescence often disrupts the concept of self. The physical, sexual, and social demands on the adolescent may produce internal conflict, an identity crisis, that requires the adolescent to develop a new self-concept. . . . Adolescents often try out different roles in the process of establishing an identity."(4) Erikson felt that the central issue for the adolescent ego was the crystallization of a sense of identity and self-continuity. In other words, the teenager must find out who he is and incorporate this with who he was in the past and who he will become in the future.

For Erikson, the developing personality passes through a sequence of eight psychosocial crises or stages in the life cycle, from infancy to old age. He called the crisis during adolescence "identity versus role confusion." He felt that his contribution in exploring the concept of ego identity would broaden rather than revise or replace Freudian theory. This particular life cycle ego crisis, for instance, corresponds to Freud's early genital stage of psychosexual development.

As part of this process, the adolescent must face the task of figuring out the role he will prepare for in the adult world. In American culture, the male in particular is required to choose a life's work. Vocational choice may cause much anxiety. Family attitudes, expectations, and traditions can increase an adolescent's anxiety. Although times and attitudes are changing, for many females identity is still dependent on marital choice and outcome. Her status and identity are often established within the role of homemaker, wife, and mother. If vocational choice is not a temporary expedient, career choice will play a more important part in role definition.(5)

The most positive outcome of the [identity] crisis is an optimal sense of identity achievement, a feeling of psychosocial well-being that results from an examination of the alternatives, followed by a commitment to one alternative within the range of possibilities. Negative outcomes include an inability to make commitments to any role, or the development of a negative identity marked by commitment to a role the individual considers bad or inappropriate.(6)

For healthy development to proceed, it is necessary for the person to experience and to incorporate into his identity both negative and positive aspects of each crisis. Each crisis is favorably resolved when the ratio of positive to negative elements incorporated into the person's identity leans toward the positive.(7)

Group Membership

Many of the doubts and uncertainties that teenagers feel are often worked out by their becoming part of a group. It is important that parents not be overly critical of their teenager's friends. The society of one's peers begins to take over the supporting role that was previously maintained by the family. Group membership mediates the transition from family member and child roles to the role of an independent, maturing adult.

This is the secret of the adolescent's tremendous dependence on the esteem and approval of his peers. The group aids the individual in establishing meaningful and healthy personal and social relationships, which entails much more than just learning to get along with people. In each other's company, they share their deepest intimate feelings and acquire the ability to know how others feel and how to respond to them in an understanding manner.

Mentors and Other Role Models

While fighting hard to separate from parents, the adolescent seeks new, warm, and understanding substitute relationships. Neighbors, teachers, and physicians can all serve as identity figures. Unlike parents, these models can be more objective and do not have to represent oppressive authority. They can often give much needed advice and help, serve as a sounding board, and bolster self-esteem, almost as a mentor. As role models, they can encourage talents and creativity and can share new hobbies and teach helpful problem-solving techniques. They can be an adult friend whom the teenager looks up to and respects. On another level, heroes, sports, and entertainment figures serve a similar function.

The Generation Gap

As today's middle-aged parents look back on their own childhood and adolescence in an effort to understand what is happening to their offspring, they find that life was simpler during the 1940s and 1950s. Entertainment involved the radio and such characters as Straight Arrow, Batman, the Green Hornet, Amos and Andy, Stella Dallas, Fibber McGee and Molly, and the Lone Ranger. Later a small black and white television brought Howdy Doody, Uncle Milty, Lucille Ball, and Ozzie and Harriet. Fun was a pinball machine, a juke box, going to the neighborhood movies on Saturday, and watching the traffic go by.

Thirty to forty years ago, high school teachers concerned themselves with their charges talking in class, chewing gum, or sneaking cigarettes. In the 1990s, they must be aware of substance abuse, child abuse, teen pregnancy, and gang warfare. It's a very different world today. Everything has changed. No longer do our neighbors keep their doors open. Teens today have to worry about drugs, sexually transmitted diseases, and a tremendous fund of technical information. Video has replaced reading. Calculators have negated the need to learn simple math. Computers have brought both simplicity and technical complexity.

Teenagers today are truly the High Tech Generation. Is it a wonder they call it a generation gap?

Parents are quick to comment, "When I was their age, things were so different." Opportunities and technology are different today. Behavior may seem more complex. However, the feelings are the same. That is the key to understanding the adolescent. When asked to describe their own adolescence, most adults are able to give a fairly accurate factual account of that period. However, their affective or emotional coloring of these memories as a rule will be absent. As a person grows older, the feeling tone associated with this developmental phase undergoes repression as he tries to forget earlier, often painful, memories and feelings. For most people, the elusive mood swings of adolescence with their accompanying feelings of isolation, loneliness, and confusion have been forgotten.

Parent–Adolescent Relationships

Parents who try to remember what it was like emotionally during adolescence will be more effective in responding to their teenagers. Parents can be a great aid to their teenagers in guiding them to full maturity. By offering interest, friendship, and understanding, they can serve as a buffer against the harsh realities of initiation into the adult world.

Emerson once wrote that there are two elements that go into the composition of friendship: truth and tenderness. Rather than offering these qualities, however, so many parents seem to fight their child's advancement toward maturity each step of the way. Due to their own problems or failings, they fail to respond to the teenager as an individual and treat him as a perpetual infant. Thus, they suppress the child's ego and stifle eventual independence. Day after day, they react only to surface aspects of behavior and fail to look underneath the fads and alliances to understand the process of maturation that is occurring.

Adolescents should be allowed to separate from their parents and find their own identity. This is not always easy if you are a caring parent who likes to jump in and help. Remember, perfection is not possible or necessary even though you care. Be yourself and your caring will shine through. Do not be afraid to set limits or tell your son or daughter how you feel about his or her behavior, both good and bad. "Tough love" is sometimes appreciated, although adolescents will seldom admit their need for control. On the other hand, they sometimes tend to rebel against all those who try to tell them what to do, confusing obedience with loss of selfhood.

Parents must change and grow also. At times it seems that the teenager is asking the parent to change completely while he will not even budge. Perplexed is the parent who hears the words, "I heard what you told me. I will think about it. But I don't promise to change." It is best to remember that adolescence is not the teenager's problem alone. It is part of the total family picture, and adjustments have to be made by all members of the family.

During early childhood, the key to parenting was to give love. During latency, it was to set limits. During adolescence, a helpful parent must learn to listen. The pitfalls to true listening are expressed in the following poem, "Listen," by an anonymous writer.

> When I ask you to listen to me and you start
> giving advice,
> you have not done what I asked.
> When I ask you to listen to me and you begin to
> tell me why
> I shouldn't feel that way, you are trampling
> on my feelings.
> When I ask you to listen to me and you feel you
> have to do
> something to solve my problems, you have failed
> me, strange
> as that may seem.
> Perhaps that's why prayer works for some people

Because
God is mute and He doesn't offer advice or try
to fix things.
He just listens and trusts you to work it out
for yourself.
So please, just listen and hear me. And if you want
to talk, wait a few minutes for your turn and I
promise I'll listen to you.

The adolescent must likewise try to understand his parents' point of view. He must realize that, in their own way, they only desire the best for him. He must realize, too, that his parents also are going through a new phase of life. Seeing one's children nearing adult status can have a profound effect on one's outlook. Suddenly, the parent is aware of middle age with its inevitable decline in biologic effectiveness, socioeconomic prestige and security, and personal flexibility. These problems combined with the individuality of the parental personality can have a great influence on the way that they see and interpret the behavior of others, particularly their own progeny.

Resolutions

The road through adolescence is long and tortuous. Many physical, intellectual, emotional, and social changes occur on the road to maturity. It is often two steps forward and one step backward. During adolescence, the rapidly growing person organizes his external, somatic, and internal realities in accordance with those of an increasingly adult world. He must learn to perform in that world and live up to adult expectations and specifications.

The manner in which they reach adulthood often appears somewhat devious. At times they may seem moody, tense, and even depressed. Sometimes, they may be as angry and emotional as the Hulk or a wicked witch. Periodically, you are amazed to see and hear a grown man or woman before you. Don't blink.

It can all change in an instant. Sometimes if we remember that the adolescent desperately wants to grow up, we can better understand and sympathize with the sometimes inadequate methods he chooses to achieve this end and the labile emotions that often accompany this transition period.

Through a maze of seemingly tangential and experimental mechanisms, he learns to cope with adult responsibility and interrelationships. This process is frightening to the adolescent. Outwardly, he assumes an adult facade, based chiefly on imitation, but within himself he knows that he teeters perilously between childhood and adult maturity.

Every aspect of his personality is driving inherently toward maturity. The inadequacy of the adolescent's ability to maintain the adult pose causes many difficulties and inconsistencies in behavior. Many times, a good deal of ground already seems to be lost because of emotional turbulence.

The teenager's entire psychodynamic system is being reorganized in order to permit him to give up childish ways and prepare for adulthood. This is a slow and difficult task, and often the adolescent vacillates between the two extremes. Some of this wavering is an expression of a very real attempt to test the unknown, followed by a return to the old, familiar patterns of childhood.

The stress and tensions of this period of life have the potential to activate earlier childhood patterns of behavior, further complicating adolescence. Eventually, however, all that seemed lost is regained, and the adolescent should move into adulthood with an enriched and reasonably stable psychodynamic system. Parents who satisfy their children's needs for comfort, love, and affection and who offer a home environment that is encouraging and helpful will do much to lessen the emotional stress present during adolescence. The buzz words for parents during this phase are "listen" and "let go."

When *both* parents and teenager try to communicate and foster an understanding of what is happening to them during this unique period of development, many of the frustrating aspects of parenthood and growing up are alleviated. Truthful is the adolescent who tells his parent, "I'm sorry if I'm not Andy Hardy." Very real is the parent who answers, "I'm not Judge Hardy either. I'm not perfect, but won't you try and understand that I'm human? I love you and am concerned about you. Maybe I can share something from my life that will help you along the way." A sense of humor also helps.

Drawing from Emerson again, it is wise to remember that "life is a series of surprises." Before long, the goal and final reward of adolescent turmoil—adult maturity—will be closer at hand. The adolescent rebel may someday produce something useful for society. In any case, he will, before long, learn to accept his individual place in life, achieve a new and different love for his parents and society, and probably go on to perpetuate the order of things by becoming a parent with a "problem adolescent" in his house.(8)

Guidelines for Success

- *Be empathic.* Remember what it was like emotionally to be the age your teenager is now experiencing. Being an adolescent involves a lot of emotional pressure and is not easy.
- *Give simple but direct answers to questions about sex and physical development.*
- *Let go.* Let them know that you are there if they need you but let them take responsibility for their own actions.
- *Offer approval.* Do not be overly negative when teens experiment with clothing fads and trends in music. Are they doing OK in school? Are they working part-time? Do they help out around the house when asked? If the answers are "yes," try to focus on the positive and not overreact.
- *Do not be critical of their friends.* Peer and group acceptance are important during adolescence.

- *Be tender and affectionate.* Do not be offended if you are rejected at times. It may be particularly difficult for your opposite-sexed teen to accept physical affection from you.
- *Set limits.* It is helpful if disciplinary limits or responses to requests come from both parents. Disagree in private. Report out a unified decision even if the message is delivered by one parent. Teens may not say it but they appreciate reasonable boundaries.
- *Listen to your teen.* This is the basis for good communication.
- *Laugh as much as you can.* A sense of humor helps reduce tension and put things in perspective.
- *Don't expect perfection.* Remember that some rebellion and turmoil is necessary for psychological growth in adolescence. Overly good teens may be constricted and rigid in their intrapsychic functioning. They may fail to develop emotionally and will show personality problems later.
- *Be consistent.* Don't waiver in your approach. This doesn't mean be stubborn. Be willing to see your teenager's point of view. Compromise where appropriate.
- *Don't give up.* Keep trying to work out your differences. Both parent and adolescent are each responsible for 50 percent of the communication problem and for 50 percent of the effort needed to find a solution.
- *Don't worry so much.* Adolescents seem to grow up in spite of all your concerns. The best thing you can do is set a good example and be a positive role model.
- *Do not be so hard on yourself.* Remember, you are human. Knowing the right thing to do does not guarantee that we will always do it perfectly. It has been shown that grown children often give their parents higher marks on parenting than you might give yourself.

This chapter has been an attempt to present some aspects of what the average teen goes through as he tries to grow up. You now have a greater awareness of the developmental tasks your adolescent is trying to complete: separating from parents, forming a stable identity, and establishing some vocational goals. You also have a greater understanding of the emotional turmoil that can ensue during this period. It is hoped this information will help you cope with all this with equanimity, listen less critically, and let go so your teen can continue to grow. There is light at the end of the tunnel, as you will see as we explore the next phase of development when we enter the world of the young adult in Chapter 5.

We are not all so lucky to have teenagers who just worry, confuse, and aggravate us. Some find major stumbling blocks along the way. Some choose coping mechanisms that impinge negatively on their lives. Others regress and fall prey to emotional disorders they cannot control. The next chapter will elaborate on some of the more serious problems and emotional health issues that can arise during adolescence.

Chapter 4

Troubled Teens

Vignette: Mark

Mark was 16 years old. He was a good student, worked after school, and played on the baseball team. He was well-liked. His teachers and schoolmates considered him a "nice guy." In spite of these positive outward signs, much turmoil was concealed inside Mark. He felt worthless and hopeless. He was having difficulty sleeping. He complained of being bored but otherwise had difficulty sharing his feelings. He daydreamed a lot. He often had stomachaches and headaches. He once told his mother, "If your life was like mine, you would commit suicide." On March 11, Mark gave his prized team jacket to his girlfriend. The next day, he cleaned his room and then cut his wrists in the bathroom.(1)

Adolescent Suicide

Mark's tragic and seemingly unpredictable death is not unique. Suicide among adolescents is becoming epidemic in the United States, where the adolescent suicide rate has tripled since 1960(2) and continues to rise. Suicide is the third leading cause of death after accidents and homicide among American teenagers aged 15 to 24 years.(3) Teenage girls attempt suicide more often, but teenage boys succeed more often. It is estimated that over 1,000 teenagers attempt to kill themselves each day, and around

18 of them succeed.(4) These statistics may be misleadingly low.
As many as 50 percent of all suicides may go unreported or
unidentified. Adolescents often disguise suicide attempts as accidents. Many single-car accidents might actually be suicides.
In addition, physicians wanting to protect families from social
stigma and shame may list the cause of death as an accident.(2)

Risk Factors

Major Depression. Depression is a major risk factor for suicide. Depression during adolescence may be accompanied by
many of the symptoms of adult clinical depression: decreased
energy; difficulty in sleeping; appetite disturbance; feelings of
guilt, loneliness, hopelessness, helplessness, and worthlessness;
difficulty thinking or concentrating; loss of sexual interest or
pleasure; feeling everything is an effort; and recurrent thoughts
of death or suicide.(5)

Signs of adolescent depression may also include crying spells,
irritability, an increase or decrease in appetite and weight, somatic complaints (e.g., headache, fatigue, stomachache, or body
pain), difficulty concentrating and making decisions, increase in
daydreams, and decline in physical appearance. Low self-esteem
may show itself through feelings of self-hatred, self-criticism, or
perfectionism.(6) Grouchiness and sulkiness are frequent.

Other Risk Factors. In addition to major depression, other
factors increase the risk for suicide among adolescents. Adolescents who attempt suicide usually have a long-standing history
of problems accentuated by a more recent acute problem, disappointment, or loss. They often lack a meaningful relationship
with another human being. Causes can include the breakup with
a boyfriend or girlfriend or the loss of an older and significant
sibling, through death or departure from the household. Peer
relationships may have terminated due to graduation or drop-
ping out of school. Other significant losses can include separa-

tion or divorce of parents, a geographical move, or a turbulent family life which lends no feeling of support or security.(7)

Prolonged and progressive family disruption, disturbed parent–child relationships, inadequate communication, physical and sexual abuse by family members, and hostile and rejecting attitudes on the part of the parents all promote suicide behavior. Adolescent suicide may be an effort at communication—a cry for help.(3)

Other personal crises, particularly those precipitated by unrealistically high expectations from self or parents, can cause feelings of failure and humiliation and lead to thoughts of suicide. Other important risk factors include psychosis, recent discharge from a psychiatric hospital, and a past history of suicide attempts or gestures. A history of a suicide attempt by a parent or other family member is a significant risk factor. Such an event lessens social restraints and justifies suicide as an acceptable solution to the adolescent's problems.(6) There may be a genetic link as well. The biological relatives of a suicide are more likely to commit suicide than adoptive relatives.(8)

Race and culture should also be considered when analyzing the risk factors for adolescent suicide. The incidence of suicide is highest among white males(4), although the rate is on the rise among minority youth over the past decade.(9) "Although whites succeed in committing suicide more often, blacks make more suicide attempts. Urban blacks of both sexes have consistently higher suicide rates than whites. Rage and violence seem to be underlying factors in this group."(3)

Sociocultural factors such as racial and ethnic discrimination, the culture of poverty, and problems related to acculturation and language influence suicidal behavior in black and Hispanic youth. Black males between 20 and 35 have a high suicide rate which seems to be related to their inability to establish vocational, racial, social, and gender-role identity during these years. On the other hand, the incidence of completed suicide for black female adolescents is consistently lower than in any other racial subgroup. This is most likely due to their closer ties to their mothers and grandmothers, who are usually strong and accessible. Hispanic females have the highest suicide attempt rate of any ethnic minority group. In spite of the high numbers, very few die because their attempts are made using low-lethal methods.(9)

The "cluster suicide" phenomenon involves the situation in which other teens attempt suicide or kill themselves after hearing about such an act on television or in the print media. These acts are not arbitrary or coincidental. The teens thus involved have gone through a similar progressive struggle with their environment. They have tried other ways, such as prior suicide attempts, the use of drugs or alcohol, and acting out through antisocial acts, to gain relief from stress and despair. The publicized suicide, by lowering inhibitions and offering a bond through identification, serves as a model for what appears to be the best solution to the adolescents' problems.(3)

Warning Signs

Prior to a suicide attempt, a disturbed teen at risk may show many warning signs. Looking back, Mark did show some of them. Studies have shown that nearly two-thirds of those adolescents who kill themselves communicated their intentions directly or indirectly to others.(10) Many have been ignored. Sixty-six to 75 percent of these individuals have visited physicians during the last four months of their life.(11)

They may show the symptoms of depression that we have noted above. There may be changes in social behavior such as withdrawal, neglect of personal appearance, an increased consumption of alcohol or drugs, an increase in daydreams, and a decline in the quality of school work. A dramatic change in behavior or personality, such as outbursts of anger, violence, or rebellious behavior, may also be a warning sign. Changes in mental behavior, including irritability, anxiety, extreme boredom, and apathy, are also important signs.

The teenager who is planning to commit suicide may also

give verbal clues such as "if your life was like mine, you would commit suicide," "I won't be a problem too much longer," or "nothing matters."

Hopelessness is the most significant danger signal of adolescent distress. If a teen feels there is no hope, he cannot envision change or conceptualize there being a solution to problems. Evidence of this attitude includes giving away prized possessions, making final arrangements, or making a will. Other signs of hopelessness include a preoccupation with death, in conversation, writing, or artwork. A sudden cheerfulness or increase in activity in a teenager previously deeply depressed may be a sign that the young person has made a resolution to commit suicide.(6) The acquisition of a weapon or other means to commit suicide should be considered a danger sign.

Teen Suicide Prevention

As a clinician, I am often asked, "How can I prevent a suicide? What can I do if I suspect that a young person I know is depressed and thinking of harming himself? What can I do to help"? There are no perfect solutions or easy answers. However, here are some techniques to think about and use.

Educate Yourself. Know the warning signs of suicide and depression in adolescents listed above and watch for them. If the symptoms last for more than two weeks, your teenager is probably showing signs of serious depression and not just adolescent moodiness. Don't wear blinders and think that it cannot happen in your family to someone you love. Look and listen for signs of distress with your whole being and not just with your eyes and ears. If your adolescent is acting differently or arousing concern, ask for help.

Communicate. Good parent–child communication is important in helping prevent suicides among teenagers.(12) It is not easy to communicate with a teenager. However, certain approaches will help your teenager to talk. Create an atmosphere of openness. Share your feelings. Admit it when you are wrong. Be empathetic and share stories about your own adolescence so that they will know that their concerns and problems are not unique. Be honest in your discussions. Avoid ultimatums and commands. Avoid being judgmental. Keeping the lines of communication open is a wonderful preventive measure. Lucky is the young person who knows that he can tell his parents and physician anything without fear of reprisal. Family support, caring, and good communication decrease some of the pressure teenagers feel and increase their inner strength.

Provide Good Parenting. Much can be done long before problems get out of hand.

> Parents of an adolescent, in general, should try to satisfy the teenager's needs for comfort, love, and affection. One is never too old for a hug or a listening ear. Parents should offer a home environment that is encouraging and helpful, full of interest, understanding, and friendship, and yet as free from overprotectiveness as possible.
>
> Adolescents should be allowed to separate from their parents and find their own identity. Peer group membership helps mediate this transition period. Remember, perfection is not possible or necessary, even though you care. Be yourself and your caring will shine through. Do not be afraid to set limits or tell your son or daughter how you feel about his or her behavior, both good and bad. "Tough love" is sometimes appreciated, although adolescents will seldom admit their need for control.(1)

Be Direct. If you sense that someone you know is thinking about suicide, do something. It is better to be wrong than sorry. Talking about suicide will not cause a person to commit suicide. In fact, it can really help to relieve the emotional pain. Reassure the person that you are there for them. Your caring and interest will help break down the isolation and alter the cycle of depression, anger, and emotional pain. Be truthful and optimistic. Don't lecture. Try to get the youngster to focus on her positive attributes. Point out that things change, but that she must be here in the future to know that this is so. Try to point out that the people in her life really need her. Emphasize that you do not feel that suicide is an acceptable way to handle problems. Try to get her to think of alternatives. Be optimistic. Tell her that you will never know what will happen by next week, but if she is dead, she will never know.

Get Help. It is hard to break a confidence. Dealing with potential suicide, however, is one time when outside help is mandatory. To show you care, you have to get help. Encourage psychiatric evaluation. The youngster may be in need of psychiatric hospitalization due to an underlying psychosis or major depression. Until some conclusions have been reached about the clinical situation, try to obtain a promise and a commitment from him that he will not try to harm himself. Sometimes ask for a written contract. Identify some people, including yourself, whom he can call if he feels suicidal. Never work alone in this situation. Set up a safety network of people who can intervene at various times and places.(12)

Encourage Therapy. Encourage both the adolescent and the parents to seek professional help. Some sources that can suggest a psychiatrist are mentioned in the last section of this chapter. Actual intervention with a suicidal adolescent can be difficult. Individual therapy here is an art that must be based on an understanding of the dynamics of this developmental phase. The key to successful therapy begins by establishing a rapport based on trust and confidentiality. If an alliance can be made, the therapist will encourage ventilation of sad feelings and activity to absorb angry tensions. Direct support with day-to-day problems in school and at home will also be discussed.

Therapy is aimed at protecting the depressed teen from harming himself, while strengthening his self-esteem. This is done in part by focusing on positive aspects of himself and his life. Even if the adolescent will not come for therapy, the parent can set an example by going for help. Their involvement in therapy may help alter the family equilibrium in a positive way. Professional intervention can do much to allay suffering, improve coping skills, and help foster growth.

There Are No Perfect Solutions. Even the best of care, attention to education, and prudent observation will not always prevent a youngster from committing suicide. Like Mark, some just do not show enough clear signs or symptoms for their underlying turmoil to be noticed even by caring parents, teachers, physicians, and friends. Often we are astonished when a "model teenager" takes his life, although studies have shown that even perfectionistic overachieving young people can be suicide victims.(8) Suicide is probably the most painful loss a family or a professional person working with a depressed patient can experience. It is particularly difficult if the victim is a teenager or young adult. We must do everything we can to educate ourselves about the warning signs of adolescent suicide so as not to overlook or minimize their importance. Threatening suicide is a warning that should never be ignored.

Masked Depression

Adolescents often do not express depression directly in adult symptoms. They may hide or disguise such feelings through a variety of behavioral or somatic manifestations in what has been called "depressive equivalents."(13) Acting out (the externalization of inner conflicts through behavior) may be signs of masked or hidden depression. Examples include behavior problems, accidents, sexual promiscuity, substance abuse, and school problems. These may also include general acts of rebellion, such as temper tantrums, disobedience, truancy, and running away from home.

"Symptoms such as boredom, restlessness, the seeking of constant stimulation, fatigue, poor concentration, and psychophysiologic reactions with hypochondriac bodily preoccupations also may stem from underlying depression."(14) Adolescents may engage in various other negative activities to escape from their unhappy thoughts. These can include fighting, verbal hostility, stealing, and vandalism. Such acting out can often be seen as conduct disorder rather than as symptoms of masked depression. Depression as a suicide risk factor can thus be missed.

Younger adolescents may deliberately deny their true feelings. This depressed youngster may pretend to be happy and show a reversal of mood in the form of a smiling depression. Older adolescents tend to express their anger more overtly through rebellious acting out and may also not appear depressed.

The adolescent tends to rebel against all those who tell him what to do because he confuses obedience with a loss of selfhood. This rebellion is an attempt to master reality, but in a regressive way. Cheating, lying, and gambling may be used as a defense against inferiority, by building up self-esteem. The high adolescent accident rate in cars, the household, and sports results from the combination of high activity and anger turned against the self. The adolescent may also act out to force the environment to provide love and care for his hopeless and helpless misery.(14) Delinquent acting out may be a "psychosocial expression"(15) of an underlying depression, which serves as a means of filling the emptiness the youngster may feel.

The sexual acting out which is seen in adolescents is often a method of relieving and escaping from depressive feelings. In this way, the person frenetically seeks contact with another human being by means of sexual intercourse, the only method of relating he knows.

A common avenue for the masked depression during adolescence is observed in the many school problems and failures which crop up at this age. College students who shift their major, interrupt their studies, attend school part time, and show prolonged indecisiveness in choosing a career may be hiding an underlying lack of self-confidence and often frank depression.(16) College students sometimes show a constellation of symptoms characterized by an apathetic state of mind which is often expressed in the phrase, "I can't make myself want to study."(17,18) Their surface blandness and paralysis constitute a facade which masks deeply repressed inner turbulence and hatred too overwhelming to be endured and bears a kinship to depression. For such students, apathy is a defense that protects them from being hurt.(14)

Substance Abuse

An American Medical Association "white paper" on Adolescent Health released in December, 1986, placed alcohol and drug abuse at the top of the list of major teenage health problems. The document noted that alcohol is the drug most often abused by teenagers and adults alike. The National Institute on Alcohol Abuse and Alcoholism (NIAAA) indicates that 20 percent of the 14- to 17-year-olds in the United States are problem drinkers. Every year 8,000 people aged 15 to 24 die in alcohol-related traffic accidents. Two-thirds of American adolescents experiment with illicit substances before they graduate from high school. Roughly one out of 16 high school seniors drinks alcoholic beverages daily.(19) Social protest and political involvement used to be hallmarks of adolescence, but alcohol and drug abuse have taken their place. Although their use could be a symptom of wanting to escape from the pressures of growing up, substance abuse is a negative position of apathy and passivity. It can certainly be a method of coping with underlying depression and a risk factor in teen suicide.

Today, those working in the field of substance abuse do not concentrate on the substance involved. Rather, they focus on the whole person because they know that addiction is a symptom reflecting psychologic stress. It is a way the teen is dealing with both internal and external pressures.

> The drug can serve different functions at different times even within the same person. It may be an attempt to deal with feelings of anxiety, guilt, anger, loneliness, inadequacy, physical pain, or depression. Sometimes, it may mask a serious underlying psychiatric illness. . . . The addict handles stress by avoiding pain and by trying to satisfy the pleasure principle. For some, it is the last grasping toward something to forestall the horrible feeling of self-disintegration or self-disorganization, which spells the doom of feeling totally helpless or out or control.(20)

It is very easy for an adolescent to become involved with drugs and alcohol. Although college administrators are setting stricter limits on the use of alcohol on campus, it is still often difficult for teens to attend a social function where beer or other alcoholic beverages are not served. Many adolescents experiment with various substances after being told by their peers, "Try it. You'll like it." Curious about the effects of such substances, they wear blinders about the possible dangers that can result from the impurities often found in nonregulated psychoactive substances. Further danger lurks if a pleasant first experience encourages continued use. If the substance starts to disrupt their lives, they have moved from experimenter to abuser. At this stage, they may turn to drugs or alcohol to complete a task or cope with a situation. Included here is the student who consumes excessive amounts of caffeine to cram for an exam, eats compulsively, or uses excessive nicotine. "Weekend escapism" would also fit in this category.

When tolerance develops or a withdrawal syndrome appears, the substance has taken over the person and her life. She has graduated to becoming an addict.

> People who become addicts have underlying emotional problems and serious unmet needs. For addicts, the effect of the substance has a specific significance. It means the fulfillment—or at least the

hope of fulfillment—of deep, basic needs. They try to use the effects of the drug to satisfy certain internal longings or needs such as sexual desire, feelings of security, and self-esteem.(20)

What Can Parents Do?

Concerned parents should ask themselves various questions and put the situation in perspective before overreacting and judging their adolescent an addict. How are they doing in school? Do they have friends? Are they concerned about others? Do they help around the house? Do they have a parttime job or a hobby? If the answers to these questions are "yes," perhaps you can lower your level of concern. Although you will not condone alcohol and drug use, understanding may help. In this day and age, many teens do experiment with substances. Turn your worry and concern into action. Increase your knowledge about substance abuse and foster education about drug and alcohol use. Are there potential risks for tolerance or physiologic and/or psychological dependence? Are there synergistic drug interactions such as those seen with alcohol and barbiturates? What are the possible side effects? Finding out and sharing the answers to these questions are a more helpful way to have your concern earn dividends.

Help is available for the teenage substance abuser on both an outpatient and inpatient basis. Alcoholics Anonymous (AA) and Narcotics Anonymous (NA) are available. Ala-Teen (for teenage children of alcoholics) and Alanon (for family members and friends of alcoholics) may be able to offer you information and support. The most difficult part of getting addicted adolescents help may be their own denial. They often minimize the situation and avoid responsibility by blaming others. "All you can do is confront them and offer empathy, love, and hope. If they don't follow through immediately, you may feel quite helpless because you care. But remember, you can only do so much. Substance abuse is a highly treatable disease."(20) When your son or daughter is ready, they will call out for help.

Eating Disorders

Vignette: Heather

Heather was referred to me by her gynecologist, who had been treating her for weight loss and menstrual irregularities. She had not had a menstrual period in two years. She was 21. All lab work proved negative. Several months prior to coming for evaluation, Heather had participated in an inpatient eating disorders program. Following this, she had been operated on for the removal of one of her ovaries. She subsequently gave up her apartment, where she had been living for almost three years, and moved back home with her parents.

The patient was thin. She weighed 85 pounds and was 5 feet 2 inches tall. She indicated that her "normal" weight was 100 pounds. She confessed that she was fearful of getting fat. She admitted that her weight had become very important to her and that she was unhappy with her body. However, initially in therapy, she denied that there was any real problem concerning her weight. Heather compulsively exercised daily to the point of exhaustion. Her self-esteem was low and she complained that she could not seem to please her parents. Like many eating disorder patients, she was perfectionistic, polite, obedient, and intelligent.

She complained of feeling keyed up and stated that she had been having difficulty sleeping for the last six months. Evaluation showed that the patient was depressed and anxious. Her appetite was poor, and there was a loss of sexual interest. Heather had been spending a lot of time worrying. She revealed that she had stopped seeing a boyfriend 18 months before, when he had been transferred to New York on business. She felt isolated. She admitted that she had had trouble being away from home but was now having difficulty living at home after several years on her own. She said that she was afraid to get involved at work because people might disapprove of her. She worried about what people would think of her.

In individual psychotherapy, the patient was able to ventilate some of her feelings about having to cope with living in her family home again and being separated from her male friend. She also dealt with *issues of self-esteem and gained some understanding of her emotional needs. She realized that she needed to feel in control. The last three years had been quite stressful. Controlling her weight had been her way of trying to regain this feeling. Individual psychotherapy along with a trial on an antidepressant agent proved successful. Heather started to eat and exercise again in a more normal manner. I knew we were going in the right direction when she started to gain a pound a week. In our last session, she reported that her menstrual period had returned. She weighed 91 pounds and was no longer afraid of gaining weight. She said that she had met and was dating an old friend and that things were better at home. My best gift came during the holiday season when a card arrived bearing the simple message, "Thanks for everything! Merry Christmas." Heather.*

What teenager is not concerned about his or her body image and personal appearance? Chaotic eating habits are typical among this age group. Food and eating are an integral part of life that help fulfill many basic needs. Food is a metabolic necessity for maintaining life. The polarities of anorexia nervosa and bulimia are the perverted extremes of this process.(21) Eating disorders may affect as many as 5 to 10 percent of adolescent girls and young women today.(22) As in Heather's case, many eating disorder patients show symptoms of depression. Recent studies report that one-third to one-half of patients with these disorders suffer from major depression.(23)

Anorexia Nervosa. Anorexia nervosa, meaning "a nervous loss of appetite," usually begins during late adolescence, with a mean age of onset of 17 years and six months.(24) Ninety-five percent of these patients are female. The disorder involves a sudden involuntary loss of all interest in eating, with marked weight loss that becomes not easily reversible. These patients show an intense fear of becoming obese as well as a disturbance of body image which causes them to claim that they are fat when in fact they may be on their way to becoming emaciated. No physical cause can usually be found to account for the weight loss. The fact that it occurs in those who are high achievers and seem to be functioning well may lead one to underestimate its seriousness. Some feel that the anorexic's compulsion to diet and her relentless pursuit of thinness develops out of a need to exert some control over an overwhelming environment and to become in some way special or unique.(25)

Bulimia Nervosa. Bulimia, meaning "hunger of an ox," is also a syndrome of food preoccupation. The disorder usually begins between 17 and 25 years of age(26), and is characterized by recurrent episodes of binge eating, usually of high-calorie, easily digestible foods. These episodes are followed by efforts to lose weight, including purging or vomiting, use of laxatives or diuretics, severely restrictive diets, or excessive exercise. Unlike anorexics, bulimics are aware that their eating patterns are abnormal and that they are under psychologic stress. They frequently suffer from guilt and feelings of helplessness and depression following binges. For some, the binging has a tranquilizing effect. Purging further releases tension, relieves the guilt of binging, calms their fear of becoming fat, and in general makes them feel better.(27)

Schizophrenia

Vignette: Paula

Paula stood at the top of the stairs and screamed. She didn't feel as if she was in control of her body or her mind. She was frightened by her image in the hall mirror. In reality, Paula was beautiful. She had a fragile doll-like quality that made her look younger than her stated age. Today, she felt that her body looked distorted. Her hair was disheveled and she thought it looked like snakes. She stood with her hands raised high over her head to stop the onslaught of terror. Her insides felt as if they were moving around. She was frightened and felt as if something was trying to harm her. She saw flashes of color that at times took on human form. It all seemed to have religious overtones.

She was sure that "they" would devour her. She heard a voice that repeated, over and over, "Kill, kill, kill." Paula didn't know whether it was God or the Devil speaking to her. She felt she had died and would be reincarnated as the Queen of Spain. She continued to scream and scream. Her agitation continued until they took her to the hospital. Paula was nineteen years old. The label was schizophrenia.

As in Paula's case, the psychotic symptoms, disorganization, and disintegration of "dementia praecox" or schizophrenia may first show themselves during late adolescence. Etymologically, dementia praecox implies an onset early in life and a loss of intellectual capacities. The term schizophrenia means a splitting of the mind. Neither definition gives an accurate description of this disorder. This psychosis is a thought disorder (in contrast to a disorder of mood as seen in the bipolar disorders). The thinking disturbance leads to difficulties in communication, in interpersonal relationships, and in reality testing. The illness varies in severity from one patient to another. Schizophrenia may really be a spectrum of illnesses or a group of related disorders. Major symptoms of schizophrenia include:

1. *Delusions*—false beliefs that are not amenable to logical persuasion.
2. *Hallucinations*—a sensory perception that occurs in the absence of a stimulus. These can be visual or auditory or involve any of the senses.
3. *Loose associations*—ideas are incomplete, fragmented, and illogical. They shift from one unrelated topic to another.
4. *Autism*—involvement with one's own thoughts to a degree that one does not relate meaningfully to any external events.
5. *Flat affect*—no range of feeling tone.
6. *Social withdrawal and isolation.*

Etiological possibilities include biological, social, and experiential factors. Although an exact cause has not been documented, most scientists conclude that schizophrenics inherit a susceptibility or genetic predisposition to the illness(28), which can be triggered by environmental influences such as viral infections, a traumatic childhood, or intense adult stress. It often emerges as the body undergoes the hormonal and physiological changes of adolescence.

At present, there is no known cure for schizophrenia. However, medications effectively control acute psychotic symptoms such as hallucinations and delusions in 80 percent of patients.(29) In conjunction with behavior therapy and psychotherapy (individual, group, and family), they can also do much to allow better functioning.

What to Do If Your Teen Needs Mental Health Treatment

Teenagers are often confusing to parents. Sudden displays of independent thought and action are often difficult for parents to reconcile. Your concern and anxiety can run rampant. Their differences in values are at times just an experiment in sorting out their identity. At times the most emphatically voiced beliefs are merely an effort to shock and test parental responses. Being able to maintain enough objectivity to gain a fair perspective is the key to success. Understanding what constitutes an average adolescent process and empathy based on remembrance of your own trials and tribulations during adolescence can help you here.

However, if communication or behavior have deteriorated to the point that they interfere with daily normal functioning, it may be time to seek professional help. It is of course best if a patient comes for help voluntarily. It says loud and clear that they want help and are willing to cooperate in treatment. It is difficult to force anyone, let alone an adolescent, to get mental health treatment. Start out by sharing your concern and caring. Show interest, understanding, and receptiveness. Present factual information and suggest that talking it over with someone objective and outside the family circle may be helpful. The family physician, who may already know the teenager and have some rapport, may be the ideal person with whom to start. If necessary, he can help facilitate a referral to a psychiatrist. Other resources to obtain a referral for psychiatric treatment include the community mental health center, general hospital, or local medical, osteopathic, or psychiatric society. Special programs are available for mood disorders, eating disorders, and substance abuse.

Even if your teenager won't go for counseling, go yourself. The perspective and information will be helpful. If you start acting differently in the situation, it will change the balance of the relationship slightly and your teen may respond differently. You will be setting an example which may have a positive effect. Teens often follow what they see you do and not what you say.

If you suspect that your teen is regressing into psychosis or if you observe the warning signs of suicide, seek consultation as soon as possible. Early intervention is important in the prognosis or outcome. Do your best but realize that professional help is necessary and useful.

One of the most frustrating situations occurs when outpatient therapy, psychiatric hospitalization, or inclusion in a drug and alcohol treatment unit is necessary but the offer of help is refused by the adolescent. Someone outside the family who has a good relationship with the teen may be able to help. For instance, seek out and enlist one of her friends to talk to her. Often, a teacher, clergyman, or other mentor for whom the adolescent has some respect and an established rapport may be able to get them to see that they have a problem and need special help. At times, gentle but firm verbal persuasion by a psychiatrist or other mental health professional can help facilitate the situation.

The teen may be embarrassed and feel guilty. Helping them verbalize these emotions and then reducing these feelings can foster perspective. Another important strategy is to reduce the adolescent's fears and anxieties about obtaining treatment and having an emotional problem. A tour of the hospital or substance abuse facility may be a way to allay such fears. Help the teenager realize that the stigma of mental illness is not what it used to be. Getting help needs to be their first priority.

At times, involuntary commitment to a psychiatric facility may be necessary. State laws differ on how this can be done. A legal and/or psychiatric opinion may be needed. Twenty years ago, in Pennsylvania, parents could place a teen in a psychiatric hospital by their own request, even out of anger or frustration. That changed in 1976. Today Pennsylvania law protects the individual's rights and prevents such arbitrary action. Anyone age 14 or older must sign in voluntarily for treatment in a psychiatric facility. Involuntary commitment is only possible if a person has been a danger to themselves or others (as shown through specific behavior) during the last thirty days. Efforts are being made to modify this law. At times, this same law makes it difficult to hospitalize an individual who truly needs professional help but refuses treatment. For instance, a depressed teen with suicidal thoughts could not be involuntarily committed in Pennsylvania unless he had tried to harm himself or someone else. Most evaluators try to take into account the seriousness of the situation when recommending involuntary treatment.

If your teenager is indeed a danger to herself or others and requires involuntary commitment to a psychiatric facility, it will be very hard for you as a parent to reach out for this help. Feelings of guilt often stand as a roadblock to good judgment. Remember, you are not placing your child in a psychiatric hospital. You are just asking for an evaluation. The physician who does the psychiatric examination and fills out the initial involuntary commitment papers will be making the final decision. In Pennsylvania, the initial observation period is five days. If additional treatment is needed and the patient continues to refuse, additional time will be requested from the court. A judge will make the decision to keep the youngster in the hospital for up to 20 more days. After this, if necessary, an additional 90 days can be requested from the court.

Although there are many troubled teens, not all will develop the serious mental health problems discussed in this chapter. Erik

Erikson(30) expected some emotional turmoil to be part of what he called the "normative crisis" of adolescence. Emotional and behavioral experimentation is necessary for growth during this transitional period. For this reason, he felt that a "psychosocial moratorium" or selective permissiveness was needed on the part of society to allow for this process. Much variation is allowable during this period of trial and error and may still come under the umbrella of "normal adolescence." However, at times, a teenager can show pathological responses to the developmental tasks of adolescence and develop the more serious emotional syndromes which we have reviewed. Professional help may at times be required to tell the difference.

It is hoped that you have not encountered any of the above problems, or if you have there has been some satisfactory resolution. Somehow, you and your adolescent have survived the teen years and he or she is about to cross over the bridge into young adulthood. Although many of the developmental tasks overlap with those of adolescence, young adulthood is also a unique transitional period that will bring new joys and new frustrations. Let's take a look at what life may be like during this stage of life.

Chapter 5

Young Adulthood
The Twentysomething Generation

Forty-eight million young Americans between the ages of 18 and 29 make up the "twentysomething generation." This group, born between 1962 and early 1970s, after the baby boomers and during a period when the U.S. birthrate decreased to half the level of its postwar peak, are also called the "baby busters." *Time* magazine(1) has characterized this generation as staying single longer and often living together before marriage. Many are "latchkey kids" who have much anger and resentment about their absentee parents. Forty percent are children of divorce. When looking for parental role models, they often focus on the approach of their more serious, conservative, and more traditional grandparents. Family life, local activism, and outdoor activities are important to them.

In the United States, because of differences in expectations as to when the youngster must take on vocational and other responsibilities, many do not develop a stable identity or obtain social maturation until the college years, or even later. Socioeconomic independence will take longer to achieve. The result is the prolongation of adolescence into a transitional period called early adulthood or postadolescence. It is a time of gradual integration during which the individual harmonizes the various components of his or her personality. Erikson called this period a "psychosocial moratorium . . . during which the individual through free role experimentation may find a niche in some section of his society, a niche which is firmly defined and yet seems to be uniquely made for him."(2)

New Anxieties and New Responsibilities

Young adulthood is a true turning point or transitional period during which people are confronted with decisions about the major adult enterprises of work, family, and marriage. There are various opinions as to the chronological boundaries of this period. I have chosen to focus on young adulthood within the framework of the twentysomething generation, extending from ages 18 to 29. Some extend this developmental period. Havighurst(3), for example, defines early adulthood as extending from 18 to 35 years of age, whereas Levinson et al.(4) include age 17 to the midlife transition at age 40 as their "middle adult era." In that we are not going to deal in any detail in this book with "the thirtysomething generation," we will allow this overlap. In a general way, much of what we will be talking about holds true regardless of the actual boundaries chosen for this period.

In any case, young adulthood is not a period of stagnation or quiescence in reference to emotional or personality growth. During this time period, your child will go from the idealism and dreams of adolescence to the reality of the adult world. He is on his way to mastering life tasks, obtaining a stable self-image, and becoming a functioning adult. Psychological development continues from adolescence into young adulthood. Many of the developmental tasks of this period overlap with those of adolescence. They include the following:

1. Developing a stable identity, including integration of personality components and a consolidation of coping style.
2. Achieving independence from parents.
3. Establishing intimacy or love relationships.

4. Establishing an occupation or life's work. Life choices and aspirations will merge with areas of competency and enable one to earn a living.
5. Making peace with parents, including integration of parental interests and attitudes.
6. Taking on social responsibility and participating in the life of the community.
7. Finding a congenial social group.

During this developmental period, individuals will have many life experiences that will cause new anxiety but also foster new responsibilities and a new behavioral and emotional maturity. These include leaving home for military service, going to school and graduating, starting work, marriage, or even childbirth and parenthood. Here during a period of experimentation, postadolescents relate with potential love objects that represent many possible combinations of choices. Gradually they start to understand their needs and the meaning of intimacy. During this time, they must also find a vocational niche and sort out many possible occupational choices. In most cases a new appreciation of parents develop as the postadolescent integrates parental characteristics, attitudes, and values.

Leaving home for the first time is a universal experience. It is an emotional event for both parent and child. In this day and age, going off to college is often the first step along the road to independence. The following will illustrate this breaking away process from the vantage point of a parent.

College Bound: A Parent's View

We all laugh and joke about looking forward to our children leaving the house so that we may have our lives back and be able to attend to our own needs. However, when the day finally comes, mixed emotions are the rule. Through a veil of tears, you say goodbye and hope that your advice and training will hold them in good stead. The days go by and you wait for the first phone call or letter. Feeling helpless, you wonder if they will be all right.

By Thanksgiving, there are tentative signs of new maturity. Upbeat messages of dorm life and new friends reach your ears. Occasionally information slips out that makes you feel that they are really learning something in their courses. Some phone calls are not so wonderful as they dump their trials and tribulations on you long distance. Worried and perplexed you wait for the next call only to find that they have forgotten it all and moved on down the road.

Christmas recess brings anxiety over grades. The envelope finally arrives. Perhaps all expectations have not been met but the grades are passing ones and life goes on. Being home again is difficult for all concerned. Four months of independence brings new attitudes, a changing identity, and a new vocabulary. Tales of parties and new friends cause feelings of trepidation. Thoughts of sexually transmitted diseases dance in your head. Can this really be your little girl or boy? Letting go is not easy. Before you know it, vacation is over and they're off once again.

It's a little easier this time to say goodbye. Emotions are still high. Spring semester brings a new verbal commitment to educational goals and promises to work harder. However, doubts and anxieties about direction and ability continue. Stories of dropped courses and dropouts fan the fire. Physical health declines and young bodies give in to lack of rest and poor eating habits. Parental concerns seem to be ignored. With warmer weather, social relationships seem to take precedence over studies. You keep your fingers crossed, set some limits, and hope for the best. Slowly you realize that you are definitely no longer in control.

The phone calls continue and its hard to gain a perspective. You listen, give advice, and share your concerns. You hang up, wondering if it will do any good. You share your feelings with other parents with college-age children and find that they also are depressed and perplexed. A letter arrives full of new insights and observations about life. Perhaps there is hope. Something good must be happening. You soon realize that growth involves moving ten steps forward often followed by two or three steps backward in a constantly shifting progression.

You continue to call and write. You send Care packages and go on with your life. The days go by and you can feel the change. A new equilibrium is developing. Even at a distance, they sound more secure and more in charge. Before you know it, final exams are here and plans are being made to return home for the summer. Talk concerns summer jobs and plans for the future.

As if in a dream, the train has reached a new station. Before you know it, they are back in your home. Bag and baggage, they return with new ideas and points of view and a new sense of self. The successes and failures of the year are placed in perspective as you hear of schoolmates who have flunked out and will not return in September. New pride surfaces as you watch their new ability to handle their needs more independently. A period of transition has passed. This has not been a year of just academics. Some emotional separation has occurred. You have all dealt with the feelings of loss. A new parent–child equilibrium has been reached. You realize that you both have grown and changed. You have both survived a rite of passage. The summer months will serve as a time to enjoy and cement your new relationship. A short respite before you both must once again move along life's path.

The initial physical separation or breaking away from the family is not always accompanied by psychological separation or individuation from parents. This is particularly true of mothers and daughters. Women at times transfer their dependence on parents to dependence on husbands. Some assume responsibility for the care of parents or siblings and remain in the parental home.(5) Even apparently intimate parent–child relationships can have many underlying reasons. Some, particularly daughters with their mothers, are close friends and confidants. Others relate on the basis of obligation and remain emotionally distant. Still others share a mutual emotional dependence.

A Place of Their Own:
A Young Adult's Perspective

For many, the initial physical separation from parents means moving to a place of their own. Moving into your own place can mean moving into your own life. Sandy represents a case in point. Let's listen to her as she describes some of her experiences during the first few weeks in her new apartment, as she becomes a consumer, handles her own finances, and struggles with loneliness and her bond with her parents.

At 22, it was not my first time on my own. However, moving into my first apartment was still exciting and scary. I had lived away at college for two years. I then moved back home for several months, started a new job, and dreamed about the future. Suddenly, the future was here. I had my own place—my own space and freedom to do whatever I wanted. It was not entirely a new experience. The new part was that I was totally responsible for myself. I had to learn to budget in a new way. I was spending only my own money that I had earned. All of a sudden I had gas, water, electric, and phone bills and rent to pay. I had to cook and clean and shop. It was not hard but it was different. I quickly learned a big lesson. If I didn't do it, it didn't get done.

There were no real worries except for being alone. The new place was quiet and peaceful. Sometimes too peaceful. There were noises and strange bumps at night. I sometimes was afraid someone would try to break in. I ate out many nights. It was a way not to be alone and I found that it was hard to cook for one. I had to find lots of activities to occupy my time. At home and at school, there had always been people around. I enjoyed running around looking for furniture and other things for my apartment. It was great getting to pick my own stuff and express myself in a place that was totally mine. For some reason, during the first several weeks, in spite of dating and seeing my friends, I found myself visiting home several times a week. Although they were often surprised to see me, my parents seemed pleased. They fed me, listened to my adventures, and gently pushed me out the door at the end of the evening. Before long, I met new people in my apartment complex and visited my parents less.

Life Choices and Other Developmental Tasks

The twentysomething young man or woman tends to explore the nature of the world accessible to them as an adult. Levinson et al., in their book *The Season's of a Man's Life* (4), talk of four major developmental tasks of early adulthood in men. These include formation of a life dream and giving it a place in the life structure, forming mentor relationships with a teacher, advisor, or sponsor, establishing an occupation, and forming love relationships by finding a mate and establishing a family of their own. When this theory was used to study women, it was found that the timing of developmental periods and developmental tasks were similar.(6) Women, however, showed greater variability completing these tasks during their twenties due to different and sometimes conflicting choices such as career versus family.(7)

Establishing an Occupation or Life's Work

A person's job is a major aspect of self-identity. An occupation is a foundation around which a life is built. "The choice of vocation—whether it is engineering or motherhood—requires the relegation of some ego models, ego ideals, possible selves, to subordinate positions. Adolescence proper is the phase during which these stratificatory processes are initiated. During late adolescence they assume a definite structure."(8) Developmental tasks tend to overlap and reinforce one another. For instance, "formulating a life's dream is central to establishing one's identity. Establishing mentor relationships with experienced adults and establishing an occupation furthers identity and facilitates independence."(5)

For women, growth in the marketplace is complicated by the issue of maternity.... For those women who choose to work outside the home during their 20's, it is a period of increasing competence and confidence, as long as the issue of having a child is in abeyance. The fear of becoming too caught up in the work world is always present for women who intend to have children.... Work, then, is confirming of one part of the women and in competition with the mothering part. For those women who become mothers and give up outside work, during the 20's, there is a tendency for confidence to be eroded because status support for motherhood as a career is lacking in the United States and because the task of motherhood is almost impossible to master.(9)

The choice of a career is a major life decision. Personality, interests, experience, and role models are four factors that determine vocational choice.(10) Propinquity or geographical location may also play a part. A significant number of young people follow in their parents' footsteps, but many are unsure of what to do and try several jobs before settling on an occupation. One of the main areas of conflict between parent and child during young adulthood, particularly between father and son, is this choice. Clinically, I remember the distraught businessman whose son chose to fix cars, the physician whose son opted to become a stockbroker, and the attorney whose offspring became an actor rather than going into the family law firm. The sons did fine and even prospered. It took the fathers some time to accept the situation and adjust.

Love Relationships

In their twenties, people move from the self-absorbed narcissism and idealization of adolescence toward a sense of intimacy in personal relationships. Initially, they may experiment and sample different kinds of relationships. During this period, self-images shift and needs change. One day postadolescents feel independent and invincible. The next day, they may feel dependent, vulnerable, and inadequate. What they need and want may change as quickly. It takes some time to really know yourself and understand your needs. Only then are you ready to form a more mature and intimate relationship. Unfortunately, most people choose a partner and start a family before they really know what they are doing or how to do it well.

Achievement of intimacy is central to the task of establishing love relationships and a family. Erik Erikson calls his sixth stage in the development of personality, "intimacy versus isolation." He describes young adulthood as the time when we must solve the "crisis of intimacy." If this effort fails, the individual may settle for highly stereotyped and formal relationships and experience a deep sense of isolation. Although having characterological problems, this type of person can be successful but will often seem like an imposter.

Erikson had in mind more than just sex when he spoke of interpersonal intimacy. He was also considering the development of "a true and mutual psychosocial intimacy with another person, be it in friendship, in erotic encounters, or in joint inspiration."(11) Intimacy requires a firmly developed sexual and personal identity. Without this, one may shy away from close relationships and/or become promiscuous.

> Intimacy involves the ability to form close and mature relationships with peers—relationships that involve more than sexual attraction. In the broadest sense, for example, intimacy may develop between persons of the same sex who share intense, meaningful experiences. The older adolescent or young adult who is incapable of forming mature, intimate relationships with others, whether in friendship or in marriage, will likely experience a sense of isolation, of being alone with no one to care for.(12)

The prize of this period is love, which is very different from infatuation. It is important for young people to learn the difference. Infatuation is a combination of idealization of the partner, sexual attraction, and sometimes much narcissism. Often full of promise that the relationship will satisfy unfulfilled needs, infatuation usually lasts about three months. A more mature love relationship, involving mutual attraction, caring, and affectionate concern, a realistic appraisal of the partner, commitment, honesty, respect, and trust, will, it is hoped, last a lifetime.

Marriage and Establishing a Family

People who marry in their late teens or early twenties often feel that they are very grown up and mature. Looking back many years later, this self-evaluation may be quite different. Many marriages during this period sometimes "fail because the narcissism of both partners produces a marriage of self-images. . . . The relationship is often the product of our internal struggles . . . very often an acting out of our adolescent images of marriage."(13) Jackson and Lederer, in their book *The Mirages of Marriage*, indicate that people of this age "like to think of themselves as being in love; but by and large the emotion they interpret as love is in reality some other emotion—often a strong sex drive, fear or, a hunger for approval."(14) Levinson says that "most men in their twenties are not ready to make an enduring inner commitment to wife and family, and they are not capable of a highly loving, sexually free, and emotionally intimate relationship."(4)

Gail Sheehy, in a section of her book *Passages*(15), which she calls "the trying twenties," lists several other reasons that young people marry. These include conforming to the shoulds of the twenties, the need for safety, the need to fill some vacancy in themselves, the need to get away from home, and the need for prestige or practicality. She also talks about the myth of the all-purpose marriage as the automatic fulfiller of all dependencies and needs. She cautions that love develops gradually and encourages acceptance of individual differences in a relationship. "The caring of experienced partners," Sheehy says, "goes less into roles and more into enhancing the special qualities and enduring idiosyncrasies that brought them together in the first place."

A good relationship, marriage or otherwise, requires work. It will not just happen by itself. A young couple needs to pay attention to three essential points. First, they must reach a mutually acceptable decision to make a commitment to grow together. Second, they must each communicate their real self, including their needs and desires. Finally, they must use conflict and anger in a constructive, creative way as the raw material for growth.(13)

Adjusting to Parenthood: Jackie and Sol

The decision to have a child effects both man and wife. Subsequent parenthood affects the lives of both parents. Having a child of your own may give you a new insight into your own parents and a new view of life. Although some men today participate more in child rearing and the running of the household, most are still primarily caught up in career decisions. Due to social expectations, child rearing has greater impacts on women than on men and may produce different crises of adjustment. Women today confront a much more complex set of possibilities and expectations. Although some opt for one or the other, most women must still decide how to juggle career and homemaker patterns.

Adjusting to parenthood, particularly to your first child, will take some time and can engender much anxiety. Let's look at Jackie and Sol as they cope with this reality.

Jackie was 27 years old. She had always been a responsible, conscientious person. After three years of marriage, she delivered her first child. A beautiful girl was born prematurely in April. Initially, Jackie had been buoyant and delighted. Every day was an adventure. However, four months later, she felt scared and lonely. At times, a sadness came over her. She found herself crying for no reason. The baby was active and seemed to be thriving. The pediatrician said she was healthy. However, Jackie worried that something bad had happened. She felt overwhelmed by the new responsibility and said, "I have to do the right thing." She waited anxiously each night for her husband, Sol, to get home from work. He was supportive and helped her with the baby, but even he was beginning to get frustrated with Jackie's behavior. Her friends empathized with her. Her mother shared with her the fact that she too had been overwhelmed at first and had even returned briefly to her parents' home. The words didn't help. Jackie continued to be fearful. Her mind kept saying, "I thought it would be so perfect . . . what is wrong with me?"

Jackie and Sol are not alone. Their feelings and experiences are universal. After nine months of anticipation and excitement, the baby is born. Hopefully, he or she is healthy and a joy to behold. You are home from the hospital. At first all is wonderful. However, the euphoria dies down and the fatigue of delivery remains. It's two o'clock in the morning and the baby is crying. The next day, you find yourself alone, without the support of spouse, parents, or colleagues at work, dealing with dirty diapers, formula and household chores.

Reality shock. This is not exactly what you expected parenthood to be like. All kinds of worries cross your mind. Will I do the right thing? Can I handle these new responsibilities? How about my spouse? Will there be time for us? Ambivalent feelings. New anxieties, fatigue, frustration, and inconvenience. These, too, are part of the panorama of being a new parent.

A new child, particularly a first child, irrevocably changes the equilibrium of your relationships and your life. Gone are the carefree days and being able to do what you want. The baby's needs will take precedence for many years to come. There also will be positive changes. The pleasure and pride of each small achievement will be great. Look in your spouse's eyes and see the love and appreciation reflected there. A newborn can give you much pleasure.

All new parents are worry warts. Beginning the task of parenting and assuming new roles is difficult and often overwhelming at first. Anxieties are increased by doubts about the ability to care adequately for the new baby. Conflicting feelings are normal. New parents need encouragement and support to build up confidence. We are not born knowing how to be a parent.

Trust your instincts. You will probably do better than you

think. A new child's needs are basic. Food and shelter and protection from harm are important to an infant. Basically, however, a child craves love, the most important ingredient in parenting. Many of the other issues will probably work out. Your initial fumbles and fears will probably cause no harm. If you and your spouse love each other, as Jackie and Sol do, your home will provide a nurturing atmosphere. A happy home is the greatest preventive medicine for avoiding many childhood problems.

Jackie and Sol have the ingredients they need to be good parents. Jackie has to lower her expectations of perfection and trust more in her natural abilities. Anxiety is a normal part of adjusting to parenthood. In all likelihood, Jackie and Sol and their daughter will be all right.(16)

A New Parental Appreciation

Another important developmental task of this period is the integration of parental interests and attitudes, particularly those of the same sexed parent. "In order to reach maturity, the young man has to make peace with his father image and the young woman with her mother image. . . . The incomplete solution of this phase-specific task can often be endured for a while until it flares up again during parenthood in relation to a child of the same sex."(8)

During postadolescence, young adults starts to humanize their parents and become aware of them as real people. They develop a new interdependence with them which involves a mutual give and take as well as a balancing of power. In conjunction with their adolescent emancipation, "children begin to recognize their parents' strengths and weaknesses as individuals who have had numerous experiences; they begin to view them in a different way. That is, they begin to accept their parents' rights, needs, and/or limitations."(10) For the first time, a parent may hear some verbalization of appreciation for having sacri-

ficed financially in paying for college or helping support them
in some other way.

The Parent–Child Bond in Young Adulthood

The parental home represents a safe haven for adolescents whether they abide by or rebel against parental authority and values. The young adult loses some of this security
and safety physically by moving away to go to school or work
and emotionally by realizing that parents are not always right
and that doing it the parents' way does not always guarantee success or safety. However, parental ties can remain healthy
and strong on both sides. The relationship can take on a new
balance based on friendship and mutual emotional support.
The young adult continues to be a significant and unique person in the parents' lives. No relationship can replace the parent–
child bond. Many will feel a sense of pride and high morale
in their children's success. Emotional ties overlap with social ties
as parent and adult child join together to uphold family traditions and celebrate holidays. Some will spend leisure and recreation time together.

Aside from spending quality time together, this period can
pay other dividends on the parental side of the equation. After
the chaotic turbulence of adolescence, it is a welcome change.
Sit back in pleasure and watch your young adult enter the workplace and gain some success. (How nice not to have to pay their
bills!) Watch with anxious anticipation as they form new relationships that seem to be building toward the future. For some,
there will be additional joys. What a delight to watch the affection of young lovers, see your son or daughter walk down
the wedding aisle, or hold your first-born grandchild. Life can
be beautiful.

Parenting is not over when your son or daughter is 18 or
21. Just as Nora in Chapter 1 remained involved and concerned
about her growing children, we continue to remain enmeshed in

their lives. The parent–child bond, formed many years ago, does not allow for complete severance of this emotional tie. Grandmothers are known to say that small children bring little problems and that older children bring bigger problems. This is even truer today. Previously, it was only those in professional and graduate schools who often could not become fully independent until late in their twenties. However, because of deficit spending and inflation, particularly in the area of housing, many young adults now stay dependent on their parents for a much longer period of time.

A 1990 *Time* magazine cover story on the twentysomething generation indicates that "the American dream is much tougher to achieve [today]. . . . Householders under the age of 25 were the only group during the 1980's to suffer a drop in income, a decline of 10%. . . . Fully 75% of young males 18 to 24 years old are still living at home, the largest proportion since the Great Depression."(1)

When a child does leave home, parental functions may decrease, but they do not disappear. Parents continue to perform a maintenance function through aid in the forms of money and gifts. Parents also continue a socialization function. Children continue to learn how to live and cope with many of life's changes and tribulations by modeling their parents. Finally, the affectional function of parents also continues. The parent–child bond is very unique and special to both parent and child.(10)

Reinforcing independence is certainly the overall theme for the twentysomething generation as your young adult child works through the various developmental tasks that we have discussed. However, there are two sides to the coin of freedom. Your home and your attention will still remain a haven against the trials and tribulations and realities of the outside world. As a parent, your job is to be supportive but not dominant or intrusive, helpful but not controlling, and most of all as loving and empathetic as you can be. The following are some guidelines to help you help your young adult navigate this period successfully.

Guidelines for Success

- *Be supportive.* Provide a supportive atmosphere for your young adult's dreams, aspirations, and interests.
- *Stop parenting as much.* Accept the fact that, by this stage, the time for teaching your child lessons is past. He or she will learn their lessons elsewhere—from books, peers, mentors, teachers, or by trial and error.
- *Teach them indirectly.* Show them by example. Continue to be a good role model.
- *Foster independence.* Encourage them to start taking on the real responsibilities of adulthood—work and earning a living, commitment to others, and taking responsibility for their actions.
- *Let them do it themselves.* Encourage autonomy. Jump in only to stand firm against clearly disastrous actions.
- *Avoid an "I told you so" attitude.* Don't be harsh if they try it their way and fail.
- *Expect some inconsistency in behavior.* There may even be some periods of regression. Maturity is usually reached by taking several steps forward and a few paces backward.
- *Take a cooperative approach to problems.* If serious problems do occur, help salvage the situation by mutual cooperation. Help them analyze what went wrong.
- *Tell your daughter her dreams are possible.* Help her break out of sex-role stereotypes and old-fashioned limits on job possibilities for women. Encourage her to go after vocational and other choices she really wants.
- *Encourage mutual respect.* Foster a relationship based on mutual respect between older and younger adults.
- *Ask for help and guidance.* Do not hesitate to seek professional help yourself and encourage it for your young adult if emotional responses during this period seem unusual or prolonged.

In spite of correct information, parental good intentions, and effort on their part, some young adults will have emotional difficulty traveling over this terrain. The years from 18 to 29 are a stressful time of life. Some develop pathological responses when they try to separate from their parents, leave home, and take on adult responsibilities. Some develop specific mental health problems. Let's take a look at the anxieties and other emotional roadblocks that can develop during young adulthood.

Chapter 6

Anxiety and Other Emotional Roadblocks in Young Adulthood

The emotional pressures of young adulthood are enormous. The twenties are a complex decade full of challenge and tension. The change and adjustment involved in gaining independence—leaving home and moving to a place of one's own, finding work and coping with financial responsibilities, and establishing new relationships—can be stressful. Emotional sequelae may result. As is true of all transitions, young adulthood is "a period of disequilibrium or flux for the individual who must adapt to a new situation, new roles, or responsibilities. Feelings of inadequacy and lack of self-confidence are predominant during transitions because of the changes that are occurring and may contribute to feelings of impatience, frustration, irritability, intolerance, and disorganization."(1)

For most, such responses are transitory and soon give way to a new integration of personality and coping mechanisms. The anxiety they feel serves a positive adaptive function, increasing alertness and effort and enhancing creativity and performance. For others, the emotional overlay of this twentysomething transitional period may engender mental health problems. Anxiety disorders may develop. Manic depressive illness, a psychosis with genetic roots, may surface. Let's look at the mental health problems that are apt to show themselves for the first time during the twenties.

Anxiety Disorders in Young Adulthood

Anxiety is the most common mental health problem in the United States today. In an anxiety disorder, the anxiety experienced is more severe, intense, and pervasive than that which we all experience as a result of the stress of everyday life. It interferes with the ability to perform or cope and thus is considered pathological or unadaptive. Four of the seven anxiety disorders—generalized anxiety disorder, panic disorder, obsessive-compulsive disorder, and social phobia—usually show themselves for the first time during young adulthood.

Generalized Anxiety Disorder (GAD)

Nancy had always been nervous. Her palms sweated on dates, and taking tests caused stomach discomfort and diarrhea. She often had difficulty sleeping and knew that she thought too much. She flushed easily, and her muscles always seemed tense and tended to ache. She was frequently restless and tired easily. Nancy was about to finish graduate school with her MBA and had been hired by Bell Atlantic. She had been looking for an apartment and planned to move out of her parents' house. She window-shopped for a new car. During the last six months everything seemed more intense. She was excited about her launch into the adult world, but she seemed to experience a persistent, uneasy, edgy feeling and was constantly concerned that everything would work out OK. She was keyed up and on edge. The knot in her stomach grew worse. She worried that she had developed an ulcer. Nancy suffered from generalized anxiety.

The age of onset of GAD varies but usually begins in the late teens, twenties, or thirties. Cognitive or psychic anxiety predominates. Its essential feature is unrealistic or excessive anxiety and worry about two or more life circumstances for six months or longer. In young adults it may take the form of anxiety, worry, and exaggerated fears about getting a job, finding a boyfriend, or health issues. Other mental aspects include feeling tense, keyed up, irritable, and nervous and shaky inside.

The anxiety also shows itself through somatic or physical symptoms. These include evidence of motor tension such as trembling, muscle tension, aches or soreness, restlessness, and easy fatigability. Autonomic hyperactivity can show itself through the symptoms of shortness of breath, palpitations, sweating or cold clammy hands, dry mouth, dizziness or lightheadedness, nausea, diarrhea or other abdominal distress, hot flushes or chills, frequent urination, and trouble swallowing or "lump in the throat." Vigilance and scanning may be evident through an exaggerated startle response, difficulty concentrating or "mind going blank," and trouble falling or staying asleep.

Generalized anxiety is a chronic phenomenon which waxes and wanes over time. The disorder sometimes seems to follow a major depressive episode. In 50 percent of patients, stressful life events are associated with the onset of the disorder and may play a role in the persistence of symptoms. Events that represent an apparent future danger or a potential loss of security are more likely to produce anxiety.(2)

Panic Disorder

The feeling was overwhelming. Ray could never remember being as frightened. He had been washing up before bed when it happened. Suddenly, out of the blue, his body was engulfed by a feeling of dread and impending doom. The sudden rush of anxiety had a crescendo effect, like waves that would not stop beating against the shore. He wanted to scream. He wanted to run and get help. He wanted to hide. But he could not focus his mind to cope with the onslaught of terror. His heart raced and seemed to want to jump out of his chest. He was short of breath and felt as if he was smothering. He tried to walk but was weak and unsteady on his feet. When he finally got to the bed, he lay there huddled and trembling, sure that he was dying or having a heart attack. He would later learn that he had just had his first panic attack.(3)

Panic disorder, the most severe and debilitating of the seven anxiety disorders, may be experienced by up to 5 percent of the population.(4) The average age of onset is in the midtwenties. We all get anxious at times, but panic disorder is different. Some describe it like being on a roller coaster ride and not wanting to be there. A panic attack is an attack of sudden and intense anxiety that comes on out of the blue. It can last for minutes or, more rarely, for hours. The attack involves a cluster of physical and psychological symptoms including palpitations, sweating, fear of losing control, dizziness or faintness, trembling or shaking, hot and cold flashes, gasping for breath, choking sensations, weakness, chest pain or discomfort, nausea or abdominal distress, numbness or tingling, feelings of unreality, fear of going crazy, and fear of dying.

Because of accompanying physical focus of the symptoms, people often seek medical attention during a panic attack. This disorder should be included in the differential diagnosis of chest pain in a young adult. Symptoms of irritable bowel syndrome in this age group also warrants ruling in the diagnosis of panic disorder.

To be diagnosed as having panic disorder, an individual must have four or more unexpected and unprovoked panic attacks in a four-week period involving at least four of the physical and emotional symptoms mentioned above. No organic factor begins or maintains the symptoms.

Panic disorder usually begins during late adolescence or early adult life, a time of choices, transition, separation, and added responsibility. "During this time, we must deal with independence, career and relationship choices, and separation from parents. It is often a time of adjustment from student or student life to full adult responsibilities. All of these issues can be complicated by unresolved dependency needs. For this reason, many have wondered whether panic disorder is related to the stress of this transitional period."(3)

Obsessive-Compulsive Disorder (OCD)

Margie was 25. She had a need to be perfect. If guests were coming to her apartment, it had to sparkle. She wanted to have everything available to fulfill their needs. However, she was glad when they left so that she could clean up. Her life was filled with anxiety, but she could usually mask it and hide it from others. She had a need to check the locks in the house and often ran back from the car to do so. She had to get out of bed several times after retiring to see if the doors were secure. Until now, none of these issues had interfered with Margie's life. Recently, she had been under much stress. There were management problems at work, her mother was sick and making more demands on her time, and her boyfriend, Dom, was having difficulty making a commitment to her about setting a date for their engagement. She felt tense and uncomfortable. Mild-mannered and passive, Margie didn't realize how angry she was. The color red took on a life of its own. She associated it with blood. It became a source of severe anxiety and fear. "I think I'm going to die if I touch anything red." She began washing her hands frequently. Margie had developed an obsessive-compulsive disorder.

OCD also tends to have its onset during the young adult years; the average age of onset is 26±14 years.(5) In this disorder, recurrent and persistent thoughts (obsessions) can give rise to a need to perform some routine or ritual (compulsion) that helps relieve the intense anxiety brought on by the obsessive thoughts. OCD can cause marked distress and interfere with normal functioning. Although patients realize that their obsessions and ritualistic behaviors are excessive, they feel powerless to stop them.

Obsessions are intrusive, unwanted, repetitive ideas, thoughts, images, or impulses that seem repugnant and senseless. They include thoughts and images of violence, contamination, sex, loss of possessions, religion, orderliness, symmetry, and doubt. The obsessive thoughts cause anxiety, which bring on compulsive repetitive rituals or behaviors. Common compulsions used to try and reduce or neutralize anxiety are cleaning and washing including handwashing, checking, counting, repeating, ordering, hoarding, touching, avoiding settings that provoke obsessive-compulsive responses, and requesting constant reassurance that the feared obsession has not occurred.

Social Phobia

Gary was very concerned. He had worked in his family company for seven years since finishing college and had done well. Although only twenty-nine, in all outward manifestations his life could be deemed a success. He was married, had two attractive children, good relationships with family and friends, a beautiful house, and a degree of financial security. His Achilles' heel was his irrational fear and discomfort of having to make a group presentation, which he avoided doing like the plague. When forced to attend business meetings, he became extremely anxious and feared sounding foolish or not being able to answer questions. He relied on memos and subordinates to relay his orders and ideas. His hands shook while writing if anyone else was around. Gary suffered from a social phobia. It was his father's seventy-fifth birthday that finally brought him into treatment. A big party was planned. As the eldest son, it was expected that Gary would give the congratulatory toast. He was scared to death to do so.

People may be afraid of many things. However, if confronting the dreaded object or situation causes severe anxiety, precipitates avoidant behavior, and interferes with functioning, a phobia has developed. Literally translated from the Greek, "phobia" means morbid "fear" or "dread." Gary had a social phobia.

Social phobias also have, on average, an early age of onset of 16±8 years,(5) and can thus surface for the first time during the twenties. The characteristic feature of this disorder is a persistent fear and intense anxiety related to a social or performance situation in which the person anticipates possible scrutiny by others or feels that he or she will do something humiliating or embarrassing. Avoidant behavior predominates and interferes significantly with daily life. A common example is being fearful of giving a speech or performing in public ("stage fright"). Other fears include the inability to urinate in public facilities or being observed while eating or writing.

Manic-Depressive Illness (Bipolar Disorder)

Anthony and Camille were married four years and had a two-and-a-half-year-old daughter. Both were 26. Anthony had been a sheet metal worker since age 19 and attended night school twice a week to upgrade his skills. Camille worked part time in a design studio. She had been dancing since grade school and still enjoyed modern dance as a form of exercise. Their lives seemed to be on the right track.

Suddenly everything changed. Camille grew progressively more depressed to the point that she ended up staying in bed for three months and not taking care of the house or their child. She had no ambition, couldn't concentrate, and was lethargic. Then suddenly, her mood changed. She grew expansive and stayed up all night planning her "career." She was sure that she was a great dancer and soon would have national acclaim. She openly flirted with the male neighbors and hugged everyone in sight. At home, she was irritable and hostile toward Tony.

Camille was very reluctant and uncooperative about getting treatment. Tony was beside himself. He felt that his life was out of control. At first, not understanding the situation, he wanted to take their daughter and leave. He spoke to a therapist and started to gain some understanding about what was happening. He went through various stages from shock and anger to acceptance. At first, he spoke only of "the illness." He admitted, "I look at the words mental illness and it makes me sad and scared." Gradually, he came to accept that his wife had a bipolar disorder. He learned that his father-in-law had suffered from depression. They worked together and were finally able to get

Camille to go for help. Lithium carbonate helped put their life back on an even keel. Things have been fine for three years.

Manic depressive illness, more recently called the bipolar disorders, has an acute onset which occurs in adolescence or early adulthood. Most commonly, as in Camille's case, the first episode is seen in the late twenties. It is not precipitated by life events but originates internally due to a chemical imbalance. There are definite genetic and familial ties. This emotional disorder is a psychosis in which the patient's reality testing and judgment are impaired. It is a disorder of mood (rather than thought as in schizophrenia). There is impairment in the ability to function. Specific psychiatric treatment is required to return the patient to premorbid functioning. The illness has a tendency to recur with multiple episodes during the patient's lifetime.

Bipolar disorder, depressed episode, will show symptoms of depression such as loss of energy, psychomotor retardation, fatigue, lethargy, decreased self-confidence, loss of initiative, feelings of helplessness and hopelessness, bodily complaints, and thoughts of death or suicide. However, the symptoms are more pronounced and extreme than those seen in other depressive disorders. They can show difficulty in thinking or concentration. The patient may complain of "slow thinking" or "mixed-up thoughts."

Bipolar disorder, manic episode, shows an elevated, high, euphoric, ecstatic mood. These patients can make you laugh. They often make inappropriate affectional and sexual overtures. There is evidence of grandiosity and increased self-esteem. This can even show itself in their choice of clothing, which may be bright colored and embellished with beads and gaudy ornaments. The emotions of such patients are labile and can quickly switch to extreme hostility and anger. They can be quite difficult to deal with. They are overactive and overproductive. They show a decreased need for sleep and often stay up all night cleaning and writing. They are easily distracted and show social intrusiveness. They experience flight of ideas or the subjective experience that their thoughts are racing.

Entering the Adult Years

It is hoped that your child will have a calmer and less emotionally eventful passage into adulthood than Nancy, Ray, Margie, and Gary did. If you do not have a family history of manic depressive illness, you will probably not have to go through Camille and Anthony's ordeal and deal with the upsetting symptoms of a bipolar disorder. However, remember, emotional growth is a gradual process. Neither behavioral or emotional maturity happen all at once. How will you know when your young adult becomes an adult? When Freud was asked what a normal person should be able to do well, he answered, "to love and to work" ("Lieben und arbeiten"). A simplistic but significant answer. The capacity to love and work truly epitomizes what it takes to complete the phase of young adulthood and enter the adult world. "When Freud said 'love,' he meant the generosity of intimacy as well as genital love; when he said love and work, he meant a general work productiveness which would not preoccupy the individual to the extent that he might lose his right or capacity to be a sexual and loving being."(6)

If one does not successfully navigate the various developmental tasks and develop a capacity to love and work, the result, usually manifested by adolescence or early adulthood, can be a personality disorder. Jay, the ferocious bear described in Chapter 2, had this problem. Genetic, constitutional, environmental, cultural, and maturational factors may all be involved in the etiology of a personality disorder.(7) These disorders are characterized by a life-long process of deeply ingrained patterns of self-defeating, maladaptive behavior. Although every area of their personalities is affected, persons with such disorders have particular problems in their capacity for work and in their interpersonal relationships. They can be intelligent and show spurts of brilliance but often cannot maintain performance because they overreact to stimuli. They have a low frustration tolerance and are oversensitive to criticism. They have trouble tolerating the emotional hurts involved in learning. They respond to setbacks at work which they bring on themselves by complaining, becoming hostile, and withdrawing.

Personality disorders are diseases of nonattachment. Those who are afflicted are unable to establish intimacy. Their relationships are shallow, weak, and stereotyped. They lack empathy, concern, or understanding, are unable to identify with others, and are involved in constant friction. They cannot forget old hurts and will bring them up years later. For them the world and its people are divided into good and bad. They lack true feelings and have been called the "empty bucket syndrome." They may complain of chronic feelings of emptiness or boredom. They often act out histrionically or psychopathically, sometimes with drug and alcohol use, in attempts to fulfill their needs and try to feel or express emotions. They often manifest no guilt feelings after acting out.

The Age Thirty Transition

In spite of all its changes and advances, the twentysomething life structure often lacks a sense of stability or permanence. Research shows that there is an age thirty transition for both men and women.(8;9) A patient of mine hinted at her awareness of this when she confided that she had started to ask people to call her Angela rather than Angie. When asked why, she responded, "I'll soon be thirty and think its time to be taken more seriously. Angela says that better than Angie."

By age 30, decisions have been made that focus the individual's life. However, Sheehy(10) again warns that at this juncture, the choices of the twenties may no longer seem appropriate. New questions are asked. Changes are made based on new choices. Commitments are altered or deepened. Levinson et al.(9) call this period the "age thirty crisis." They indicate that this transition, occurring between ages 28 and 33, allows men a second opportunity for establishing a life structure more congruent with the life dream. For some, this period takes on a sense of urgency, and they start to feel that issues must be addressed quickly because it will soon be too late to make major changes.

In any case, by the early thirties, both parents and child are in a different place both within themselves and with each other. Although they will henceforth relate to each other as two adults, the parent–child bond will continue to evolve. During the twenty-something decade, the child leaves home, begins an independent life style, achieves occupational goals, forms new relationships, and sometimes starts a family of his or her own. However, parent and child continue to be significant people in each other's lives. Emotional, affectional, and social ties continue. They may join together to uphold family traditions or celebrate holidays. Although they may maintain "intimacy at a distance,"(11) by having separate homes, many want the assurance that they will have someone to depend on when they need help. As time goes by, "the interactive drama that began with conception continues . . . with new plots, but with old characters and old relationships still evolving and unfolding."(12)

In the last four chapters, we have looked at what your children have been doing between the ages of 13 and 30. We have examined their problems, their dynamics, and some of their resolutions. It was our hope that this information would enable you to stand back and look at the big picture and be better able to evaluate what is happening in your child's life during these stages. Now, let's take a look at you, the middle-aged parent. Parents can have problems, too. Let's see what is going on with your generation as you try to cope and interact with your growing children. During these years, you may be fighting your own battles. They may have nothing to do with the adolescent or young adult issues at hand, but they certainly do complicate the picture.

Part III

THE SANDWICH GENERATION

Chapter 7

The Challenge
of Middle Age

Vignette: Rob

Rob moved slowly down the theater aisle, oblivious to the crush of people around him. The strains of the song "Diana" continued to reverberate inside him. Hearing Paul Anka's songs of the fifties once again, with their throbbing surge of adolescent hormones and simplistic, idealistic messages, had made him feel 30 years younger. In his mind, Rob could see himself as a young man, thin, vibrant and agile, dancing to these fifties tunes. All at once, he was filled with emotion and thoughts of the past and the future.

Rob was 48 years old and married, with two young adult children. Long ago, he had left behind the dreams of youth and concentrated on the more realistic goals of adulthood. Everyone would deem his life successful, and yet he suddenly wondered if that's all there was. His mother had died last year, his father was developing cataracts, and his wife was wrapped up in her own career. His children were going in their own direction. The dog had died in the spring. Rob suddenly realized that he also was clearly enmeshed in middle age.

This sudden pull backward in time filled him with a sense of melancholy. He was surprised at his own strong feelings. Rob was very aware of the stations he had passed in his train ride through life. It was more than half over. For the most part, he was content and felt

*that he had done well. However, for a moment, he felt very fragile and
vulnerable. Where did he go from here?*

*As he drove home from the theater, he continued to think. There
were so many things he wanted to do. He would never be a young
man again. To make matters worse, there never seemed to be enough
time. His children, although out of the house, still leaned heavily on
him and his wife for both emotional and financial support. His father
and widowed mother-in-law were getting older. Their health was declining and they seemed to need Rob and his wife more. For a moment,
he felt frustrated and angry. "When will we have time for us and be
able to do what we want?"*

Rob is not alone. The ranks of the middle-aged are increasing. "Today, there are more than 50 million men and women in
the United States—one-quarter of the total population—who are
in the midlife period from age 40 to 60."(1) The musical decade
of the fifties, which inspired Rob's reverie above, along with its
pastel colors and T-Bird cars, has turned forty. The baby boomers
are moving into middle age. Hank Ketcham's cartoon, Dennis
the Menace, also has already had its fortieth birthday. Believe it
or not, "That pint-sized hurricane . . . has been tearing through
his suburban turf and terrorizing neighbor Mr. Wilson since 1950.
And the forever 5½-year-old baby boomer shows no signs of
slowing in middle-age."(2) In 1990, Bugs Bunny turned fifty as
Warner Brothers celebrated the golden anniversary of the cartoon
star's first starring role in "A Wild Hare," which premiered on
July 27, 1940.

The Middle-Age Dilemma

Robert's feelings and internal struggle are not unique. Many
of you, members of the Sandwich Generation, will experience
high levels of stress and confusion (and often guilt) as you try
to deal with your own needs, the demands of those around you
in the family structure, and your newly awakened midlife anx-

ieties. Caught between generations and responsibilities—this is the middle age dilemma.

Middle age is a developmental phase with specific tasks and various possible resolutions. It is a time of reassessment of life goals, a time of change and conflict, which affects both men and women. It has been popularized as the "midlife crisis," beautifully defined by Darrell Sifford as "the nagging pain of unfulfilled dreams and the agonizing confrontation with discrepancy—facing squarely the gap between how we thought our lives were going to be when we planned them and how we now know they really are.... A time when we begin to see life as it really is—full of its ups and downs."(3) This process is also part of the middle-age dilemma.

Middle age can start at any age (usually between 35 and 50). It is a state of mind rather than a specific chronological age.

> Midlife or the climacterium is often seen as a time when men and women, having resolved the conflicts of adolescence and made the important vocational and relationship decisions of young adulthood, reach a period of calm and maturity. This is not always the case. The years from 40 to 60 can also be a time of change and possible conflict. During this time, men and women confront physical and psychologic changes which cannot be ignored. You also may confront an assortment of life stresses and must adjust to the prospect of aging. All of this can cause crisis and upheaval for some. For others, it can be a time to reintegrate biologic, psychologic, and social components and establish a new balance. It can be a time to crystallize a self-concept, heighten creativity, and increase productiveness. Lastly, it can serve as a bridge to prepare a person for old age.(4)

What happens during middle age that creates the turbulence and agitation that some experience as a midlife crisis? Maybe it's due to hormonal or physical changes. Maybe it's an emotional change borne of a growing awareness of mortality—a sense that time is running out and that you are more than half way through this play called life. Maybe it's a combination of both factors. Regardless of etiology, the energy of this phase can be used constructively to build on what you already have. Or it can be used destructively to breakdown and throw away your past. This is the choice.

Midlife is a time to look backward and reevaluate and reassess earlier decisions and patterns. It is also a time to look forward to the future. This unknown can be dark and scary. It can intimidate you and cause you to withdraw and stagnate. Or it can be seen as a challenge, a time to take charge of your life and move forward toward more success, accomplishment, and contentment in the future. Many myths need to be recognized and dispelled to really understand and deal with this stage of life more constructively. Let's look at some of the critical issues that impinge on men and women during this time.

Menopause: A Time of Change

An elaborate mythology suggests that women go crazy during the change of life.(5) However, change of life is not a sickness. The climacteric is a universal phenomenon(6)—a normal process through which all women (and men) pass—a natural phase of life. (The terms climacterium and menopause are used by some interchangeably. The term menopause has a restricted connotation meaning the cessation of menstruation in the female.)

Some feel that the menopausal syndrome is largely a social role foisted on middle-aged women by American society. They also feel that the physician (usually male) plays an inadvertent but active part in recruiting women into this role.(7) Much of the anxiety about change of life is due not to its actual physiologic effects but to the deep-rooted, negative attitudes we have toward aging in the United States. In cultures where the elderly are revered—in China, for example—change of life produces little psychologic concern.

The waning of ovarian function and the cessation of menses usher in an epoch that endures to the end of a woman's life.

Some go through a difficult time, but the majority need not have any difficulty. The changes that occur during this time of life are related to a rebalancing of physical, hormonal, and chemical patterns for the female.(8)

There are certain symptoms that may be caused by the various hormonal changes that can take place during this stage of life. (There is usually a decrease in estrogen and an increase in luteinizing hormone and gonadotropin.) These include a vasomotor imbalance with hot flashes and increased perspiration and physical changes, such as atrophic vaginitis and other signs of urogenital-tissue atrophy leading to dysuria (painful or difficult urination) and urinary stress incontinence. Other physical symptoms include palpitations, migrainoid headaches, and bone degeneration.

There can be emotional symptoms such as fatigue, depression with feelings of futility and uselessness, insomnia, anxiety and nervousness, and sexual dysfunction.(9) A woman may express change through irritability, hypersensitivity, excessive complaints, or multiple somatic symptoms.(10)

Middle age can present a life crisis just as earlier or later developmental phases do.(11) The adjustment, however, depends as elsewhere on general adjustment of the personality and the ability to take a problem-solving approach to life. It is an event of psychologic significance, particularly for the unfulfilled.(12)

There are connections between menopausal reactions and the woman's attitudes about her menarche and menstrual cycle, her feelings and conflicts about sexuality and femininity, and her relationships and identification with her own mother.(11) The woman's attitude toward this gradual decline in her reproductive capacity draws on many early fears reinforced by her concerns that she will be less attractive to her spouse or as a woman.(10) She fears that she will be abandoned and become old and purposeless.

It has been found that women who report a higher number of menopausal symptoms tend to be less well-educated, are less likely to be working, and view themselves in poorer health than women with fewer or no symptoms. It has also been found that symptoms such as depression, headaches, and irritability were found to be significantly related to personality attributes such as self-confidence, personal adjustment, nurturance, and aggression.(13) Overweight women, compared to other women, seemed to suffer less "somatic" (bodily) symptoms, such as hot flashes and perspiration (possibly as a consequence of the higher endogenous estrogen activity). On the other hand, "emotional" symptoms such as anxiety, depression, irritability, and crying spells seemed to be more frequent and more severe in the obese group. (Most likely these symptoms were due to psychosocial factors.)(14)

The Male Climacteric: Middle-Age Crazy

Problems during middle age are classically seen as a female issue often attributed to menopause. However, at this age, men also may be forced to come to terms with the fact that they are getting older, that their looks as well as their physical and sexual vigor may be changing. We are coming to realize that just as women go through menopause and a midlife developmental stage, men may experience, at approximately the same age, a "male menopause" or climacteric. This current awareness may be due to the fact that more men now live to reach the period of life from ages 40 to 60 when a general slowing of physical processes may be expected. It may also be more apparent because we are living at a time when sex-associated difficulties have become more acceptable to talk about.

As in the female, the exact relationship between hormonal change in the male and climacteric symptoms is debatable. However, we do know that reduced secretion of testicular hormone is a normal part of aging. Most commonly between ages 48 and 60, pituitary gonadotroinic hormones are increased and testosterone levels are decreased. However, the fallacy that many men believe is that there has to be a sexual decline after age 50. Age does bring some modification in sexual responsiveness. Older men achieve erection more slowly, just as women may have a reduction in the number of orgasmic contractions, but do not necessarily show a decline in desire or pleasure.

Physical illness such as diabetes and therapeutic medications such as antihypertensive agents can influence sexual potency. However, once normal age-related physiologic changes in response patterns are recognized and understood, continuation of satisfactory sexual activity in otherwise healthy males is to be expected.

The male climacterium, as in the female process, may be marked by a variety of emotional symptoms, including depression, a sense of frustration, disillusionment with old goals, and a sudden awareness that "time is running out." These feelings, if recognized and understood, may be extremely useful motivational forces leading men in middle life to adapt new, productive, more creative and satisfying living patterns. Without such recognition, they may succumb to overwhelming feelings of anxiety and react to the crisis by changing everything around them.(4)

> Under biologic, psychologic, and cultural pressure, the middle-aged man may suddenly plunge into sexual escapades with younger women or make desperate changes in lifestyle because of a feeling that life should have more meaning than it does. New marriages, new values, new jobs, cosmetic surgery, and drug experiences are not uncommon—anything to help him forget or ignore what he is actually experiencing.(15)

Unfortunately, many do not come for help until after they have burnt their bridges.

Theories of Middle Age

Like other transitional periods, midlife has various developmental tasks(16) that need to be addressed. Although specific issues differ from person to person, all of you will probably struggle with some of these matters. During this time, men and women become concerned with doing something useful in life. This may involve creativity, community responsibility, and, most important, guiding the next generation. You will also involve yourself with maintaining your occupation and your income, relating successfully to your spouse or significant other and your family, and maintaining and developing recreational activities and social contacts.

Feeling less burdened by the pressure of the goals and responsibilities of young adulthood and the stressful career and family-oriented productive thirties, some may change direction and emphasis. Men may start to reach out more and focus on relationships. This can mean new interests and new friendships. At the same time some women may just be starting their career phase. Both men and women will start to develop a deeper sensitivity to the needs of others. You may be slowed down a bit in your efforts by the two threats to midlife adjustment—middle-age fatigue and middle-age discontent. You will be forced to come to terms with the physiological and emotional changes of middle age, your own aging, and the aging of your parents. You will have to face your own mortality. Let's look at some of the psychological theories of middle age in an effort to understand these tasks and some of the things that are helpful to do to make a smooth transition through this period.

Sigmund Freud. Classical psychoanalysis, stressing the influence of childhood on psychic life, considered development to be restricted to the early years. He felt that adult psychopathology is caused by pathogenic thoughts and feelings that could be traced first to childhood trauma and later to childhood fantasies. The psychoanalytic theory of development, the libido theory, is a theory of childhood development. Psychoanalysis has only recently started to embrace the whole life cycle and to try to extend its model of development into middle age and beyond. Let's see what some others after Freud had to say about the dynamics of middle age.

Carl Jung. Jung, a psychiatrist and a member of Freud's inner circle, founded a school of psychotherapy called "analytic psychology." He was the first to propose the distinction between the first and the second half of life, with the years around 40 as the meridian. Jung felt that the early stages of development were devoted to strengthening the ego (a subdivision of the mental apparatus) and establishing coping mechanisms to deal with the external world. The developmental task of the second half of life, middlescence, beginning at about age 40 and continuing through the remaining years of life, is devoted to achieving a new integration of the personality and discovering the inner, true, or real self. He called this process "individuation." Its goal, which may never be achieved, is "self-realization," or the evolution of one's unique full human potential.

During a successful process of individuation, the mature adult achieves a self-realization in which the "collective unconscious" (the inherited possibilities of form and functioning universal for all humankind) reveals the accumulated wisdom and experience of human existence. This may involve taking new paths that can be in opposition to your prior ideological position in life. The change often leads to broader more mature relationships and to an inner creativity.(17,18)

Eric H. Erikson. Erikson expanded on Freudian psychology. His well-known "eight stages of man" extended, for the first time, the concept of development throughout the life cycle. Adolescent turmoil involved the question "Who am I?" Midlife asks the question "What am I doing?" A good answer can involve making a commitment to care for and guide others. In this way, we pay back the world for what it has given us. Improving life conditions for future generations can be a primary task in midlife. This can include serving as a mentor for the next generation or helping the multitude of people desperate for care and attention. Such a choice will pay dividends for the rest of your life. Erikson(19) describes this, his seventh stage of personality development, as the crisis of "generativity vs. stagnation." He felt that if you could not invest yourself in and provide direction for the next generation, then you would fall into a mode of self-absorption concerned only with your own needs and desires.

Erikson felt that the central focus of generativity and the main goal of midlife was to be productive and creative. Wide variation is possible here. Contributing time and talent to charities, serving as an advisor to institutional boards, or participation on school and church or synagogue committees can serve this function. "By achieving a sense of generativity, middle-aged adults develop the skills to make decisions, plan for the future, anticipate others' needs, and make a purposeful impact upon the future."(20)

Stagnation, the opposite pole of the crisis, produces interpersonal impoverishment, a sense of personal deficit, and a productive failure. Here the person feels that he or she is on a meaningless treadmill expending a lot of effort but going nowhere(21). Self-absorbed adults will be involved only with their own needs, perhaps spending their efforts questing toward wealth or youthful appearance. Erikson did not mean for these two outcomes—generativity and stagnation—to be mutually exclusive. Healthy development requires that the person experience and incorporate into his or her identity both negative and positive aspects of the crisis. A favorable resolution involves a ratio which leans toward generativity.(22)

Middle-aged women who have been homebound and family-oriented may have difficulty in midlife. They may not know what to do with their new free time when their children leave home and may lack the skills necessary to contribute in the community or begin a job. (See Chapter 8.)

Daniel J. Levinson. This Yale researcher and his colleagues reported on their work on the stages of development for adult males in 1978. Their book, *The Seasons of a Man's Life*(23), stresses the fact that development is a continuing process. Their model of the male life structure involves three major eras: early adult (17–40); middle adulthood (40–60); and late adulthood (60+). During a midlife transition, men modify and reappraise the past, explore new possibilities both in themselves and in the world, and create a new structure for the future. This is done through the developmental process called "individuation" (see Jung above). This refers to the changes in a person's relationship to himself and to the external world.

Levinson speaks of various developmental tasks during middle adulthood. He says that a man must modify or give up "The Dream" formulated during early adulthood. In reference to work, having come up the occupational ladder, he now must make a place for himself in the middle adult generation and become "senior" within that world. In reference to relationships, the middle-aged male gets in touch with the feminine in himself and others and becomes more interested in mentoring his children and others and supporting his wife's need to expand outside the family.

Men during this time tend to question every aspect of their lives and focus on what they have done and what they have accomplished. Participants in Levinson's longitudinal study began to fear in middle adulthood that they would not be able to express some aspects of their personalities. From this period of questioning, a new life structure should emerge. For some it will mean continuing as before but with a new sense of commitment, enthusiasm, and fulfillment. For others, there may be changes in career, marriage, or life style.

"The stages of a woman's life used to be marked primarily by her capacity to reproduce. One critical stage came at puberty, marked by the onset of menstruation, and the other at menopause, marked by the end of menstruation and the capacity to bear children. Women today confront a much more complex set of possibilities and expectations. As work becomes central for more women, their crises of adjustment may come more closely to resemble those of men."(1)

Abraham Maslow. This twentieth-century psychologist focused on the needs, development, and maintenance of a healthy, well-functioning personality. He developed a hierarchical organization of human needs which he felt motivated our behavior. He included four levels of needs. First are the basic or instinctual needs such as hunger and thirst. Second are the deficiency needs (D-needs) such as self-esteem, love, and belonging that maintain a stable, secure individual. The next level are the B-needs or growth-oriented needs such as the need for truth, beauty, and individuality. The fourth level of needs in the hierarchy is the need for self-actualization or the achievement of one's complete potential. The highest level is the desire for self-transcendence. Here B-needs become so important that people are willing to forego basic needs to achieve higher goals.

Maslow felt that the purpose of life was to shift the balance from D-needs to B-needs. The culmination of a balanced approach to life is self-actualization. We approach closer to psychological health as we become more our real selves and less the persons we expect others want us to be. "Self-actualized people are described as realistically oriented, spontaneous, problem-centered, creative, independent, and generally accepting of themselves and others."(24) What a wonderful goal for midlife—to achieve better integration of our personality or self-actualization. Although Maslow does not specifically focus just on middle age, we include his basic concepts here because of their intrinsic value in conceptualizing a holistic view of the psychology of midlife.

Guidelines for Success

All of these theories of middle-age development appear to have one central theme—growth of the personality in the direction of achieving one's full potential, whether it be through achieving Erikson's generativity or working toward the self-actualization of Jung or Maslow. Although none of these theorists believe that we can achieve perfection, they all appear to encourage the blossoming of the personality during middle age. I certainly agree. The sense I try to communicate to my patients is that middle age is a positive time—another chance to grow. It is a time to pay attention to the quality of life. It is a time to build and expand on the gains of prior developmental periods. It is another opportunity to work through failures and unresolved problems. It is a time to go back and pick up the pieces of the puzzle that you had to leave behind in order to focus your energy on education, work, and child care. Here are some areas to focus on and some possible goals to achieve.

• *Self-Improvement.* Continue to work on yourself. Be yourself. Drop the facade of trying to influence, impress, please or win applause. Accept yourself and try not to be so hard on yourself. You have gotten this far. You must be doing something right. Accept others and stop trying to change them. Although it is true that we often expect perfection from those we care for, it is helpful to not expect so much. In reference to the adults in your life, remember that someone else already trained them a long time ago. You can't control others. You can only control what you do. Approaching life without the anxieties of youth and the compulsive pressure of early adulthood can be just as rewarding and even fun.

• *Relaxation and Recreation.* Develop new interests and broaden your horizons. Try new things and explore new avenues. Investigate new hobbies, sports, or philanthropic interests. Gain additional education. Reach back and take up an old hobby or indulge yourself in things that used to bring you pleasure before you got on the treadmill of life. Relax. Take some time just for you and leave your self open for new ideas. Take a "mental health day" off from work from time to time. Give yourself a few hours each week just to follow your nose and do whatever you want to do. You will particularly appreciate this when you decide to retire. Many have a difficult time in retirement because, having devoted themselves only to work, they do not know what to do with themselves at leisure.

- *Relationships.* Foster new friendships and deepen old relationships. Men particularly seem to have few intimate, nonsexual friendships. Midlife is a good time to rethink your priorities and try to reach out more to others. Middle age is a time to get to know people of all generations: they all have something to offer. It is also the time to work through old relationship issues and leave behind old feelings of resentment, anger, and hurt. Many people hold on to these conflicts, particularly with their parents, as a way to avoid growing up. As long as you are enmeshed in old squabbles you don't have to move on or deal with new issues and the future.

Psychologist John Bradshaw, in his crusade to help the adult children of dysfunctional families, instructs his charges to treat and heal the hurt child they carry within. I would add that it is also important and possible in middle age to go back home, repair the damage, and continue to work on parental and family relationships. As an adult, perhaps armed with new insights and understanding, you may be able to see the broader picture, forgive them and yourself, and find something positive in these relationships.

- *Work.* Do not neglect your work. Satisfaction in your job can also lead to generativity. Be available to teach younger colleagues and pass on your knowledge and skills. If you are receiving some sense of fulfillment from your occupation, it is usually best to build on what you have. However, this does not mean that you cannot develop new avenues in your employment or encourage new avocations. Seek out new projects and work toward new accomplishments. Be creative and remain productive. Share your talents and expertise. Be available as a mentor to the younger people in your field.

The challenge of middle age is personal growth—to stretch yourself behaviorally and emotionally—to grow up and continue to expand in every dimension toward your full mature potential.

You never know what will happen unless you try. Remember, as Emerson said, "Life is a series of surprises."

"The climacterium, like adolescence, can be a period of emotional turbulence. However, if navigated successfully, it can be a stage of new integration and more creative productivity. It can bring a [new] sense of self and prepare you for growing older in comfort and contentment."(4) People achieve different degrees of life success in middle age. Some achieve personal growth and others stay mired in loneliness and discontent, consumed by boredom. Some have major difficulties in their marital and other relationships and in their job satisfaction. The next chapter will deal with some of these crisis points in middle age.

Chapter 8

Crisis Points in Middle Age

Vignette: The Jolly Roger Syndrome

The evening cruise was billed as a delightful night under the stars. It turned out to be much more. The water was calm. The old sailing vessel moved slowly through the Gulf of Mexico. The crowd of approximately two dozen couples of different ages and nationalities spoke quietly to each other in small groups and drank the pink and white rum drinks served in plastic cups. Everyone relaxed. We had three hosts—a middle-aged man and a young woman and man both in their twenties. All three wore authentic pirate costumes complete with knee-high black boots and daggers.

As the sun set, the music seemed to grow louder and our older host more active. He grew more visibly tense. He quickly moved from couple to couple, talked to each of us, danced suggestively with each of the ladies, and tried very hard to appear as if he were having fun. He made a big point of telling us that he had left his stressful life behind. As the evening progressed, we gradually pieced together his story.

John was 45 years old. He had been an executive in a large Silicon Valley company, where he worked 12 to 14 hours a day. At 42, he had reached the top of the corporate ladder and was named president of the firm. That same year, he had his first heart attack. Although the attack was mild, he was scared to the core. Within six months, John sold his home and moved his wife and three children to an island town. Here he bought an old ship, The Jolly Roger, and started a new business of entertaining tourists. His family was discontent with this vagabond life. After six months of arguments and futile attempts to get John to rethink his decision to change everything in his life just for the sake of change, his family said goodbye and moved back to California. John now lived with Jan, our 25-year-old hostess.

John hurried back and forth from one end of the ship to the other, giving orders, and generally making a fool of himself. Halfway through the evening, he climbed onto the side of the ship and screamed, "Which of you women stuffed up my toilets?" Joey, who we now knew was the first mate, dropped a tray of hors d'oeuvres. John later announced that one of the motors was broken. His tension level continued to rise. It was hard to believe that anything had changed in his life except for the geography. As an adult, you can't escape responsibility. John left the corporate world behind only to find new responsibilities in paradise.

There are many middle-aged men like John. Propelled by inner anxiety and turmoil, they make destructive choices in mid-life, deciding to change everything around them, perhaps trying to deny their mortality and hold back Father Time. Trying to give life more meaning, they look in all the wrong places for intimacy, peace, and happiness. Feeling they are running out of time, they race from bow to stern trying to fulfill adolescent dreams and unwilling to face the gap between their expectations and reality. They may work even harder, have affairs with younger women, destroy their marriages, become involved with substance abuse, change jobs and locations without forethought, overdo exercise and health fads, have unneeded cosmetic surgery, go on buying sprees, or take undue financial risks. They may go on one vacation after another. I call this extreme reaction to midlife the Jolly Roger Syndrome.

All people do not react in midlife in the extreme way that John did. However, most do reevaluate their lives and goals sometimes during middle age. No one's life is perfect. Each man and woman must somehow confront the discrepancy between what they thought life would be and how it actually turned out. There are all degrees of midlife distress. Although we all go through a midlife transition, there is not always one tumultuous emotional upheaval or crisis. Sometimes the various issues are dealt with piecemeal at different times. However, during midlife, it is not uncommon to reconcile personal, relationship, and occupational goals. Let's look at some of these issues and some of the age-specific stresses that can cause problems during this transitional period.

Stress in the Marketplace

Work changes are significant life stressors at any age. At midlife, they are even more traumatic. Layoffs, stalled promotions, disappointing raises, and today's general economic uncertainties play havoc with middle-aged budgets trying to cover college costs, perhaps lend a hand to an aging parent who requires extra medical care or nursing home placement, and put aside some money for the future and retirement. As companies downsize as a hedge against recession, job loss and the threat of job loss become potent causes of stress in the workplace. Middle-aged workers may be the first to be laid off or be offered early retirement. Such corporate restructuring has made mid-career redirection much more common. Harry S. Truman said that it's a recession when your neighbor loses his job; it's a depression when you lose your own. This is certainly true financially and emotionally.

Being unemployed is unpleasant at any age. In midlife it is both upsetting and frightening. Sending out resumes and going for job interviews at age 45 or 55, for instance, is stressful and sometimes demeaning. Uncertain about their ability to once again find a job, or compete with younger colleagues in the job market, the middle-aged male or female may be filled with anxiety, frustration, anger, and guilt. This may translate to irritability, depression, somatic complaints, and even sexual impotence. If not nipped in the bud, either by increased emotional support from family, friends, or therapist, these feelings can quickly spiral downward into the dark abyss of depression.

Family tensions increase as the days of unemployment continue. Arguments over finances can escalate. Money in a marriage is often a train that people use to send messages back and forth to each other concerning other needs. As the tensions rise in the individual and in the household, arguments may become more common. The individual, used to feeling needed and in control, may start to feel unappreciated, lonely, unworthy, insecure, and out of control.

In your twenties, you thought that you could do anything. The path seemed very clear. At midlife, you may have to face the realities of the marketplace and of your own abilities and limitations. You may have to realize that you may never fulfill your potential or that perhaps the potential never existed. During this time, there can be anxiety and turmoil related to occupational life. Although work is important for income, it also serves as a source of identity, of a sense of accomplishment, and of self-esteem. As the likelihood of promotions and salary increases become slim, frustration and painful reevaluation can diminish self-esteem. Some find that they feel trapped, bored, and unhappy at work. Often they cannot go any further in their jobs and complain of repetitiveness in their lives. Some are still trying to answer the question, "What am I going to do when I grow up?" If they cannot readjust the dream of an idealized self or make appropriate career changes, feelings of depression may result.

A special situation which I have seen in doing therapy is the man who thinks he went into a profession, job, or family business due to family pressure. Here, even in midlife, there may still be much ambivalence and regret about occupational choice. Such was the case of Barry Lewis.

Vignette: Barry

Heir to a large East Coast retail business, Barry was never sure what he really wanted to do vocationally. He graduated from college as an accounting/business major and worked for the family corporation for several years. In his late twenties, he suddenly moved to California and took a job with another business. After two years, Barry left California, returned to the East Coast, and rejoined the family business. Now in his forties, he still spoke of his dissatisfaction with his work, doubts about his own abilities, and his problems with his father. He was particularly upset because he had not taken more risks earlier in life. In therapy, Barry was able to resolve old issues and make some peace with his father. He still fantasized and spoke about alternative businesses, franchises, and consulting work he would like to do. However, nothing changed. He never put his ideas into action.

A year later, his father died and Barry returned for additional therapy sessions. At about the same time, he was given the opportunity to be bought out by another firm. It was as if his dream had been answered. However, his indecision continued; he ruminated, agonized, and struggled over his choices. In therapy, he was able to understand that part of the reason he had stayed with the family business initially had been the basic financial and emotional security it offered. Now, he struggled for the first time with standing alone emotionally. He realized that although he always saw his father as a potential source of support, he had never really leaned on him. In fact, he had been making good independent business decisions for many years.

The other issue that troubled Barry had to do with his identity. Although successful, he never felt he was his own man professionally. However, he gradually began to realize and accept that he had been in business for many years, was well respected in the business community, and was seen quite differently by others. He started to feel more secure and better about himself. He finally decided to make use of his resources and expertise and stay in the same business. He worked out a parttime position with the new firm and started his own consulting firm in the same field. He seemed much more content with himself and his work.

Even successful middle-aged individuals struggle with career issues. They too must make the choice to fight, take flight, or settle for stalemate. Now that the financial goals have been reached, he or she may still be left with a feeling of "Is that all there is?" However, because of the long period of training and emotional and financial investment involved in the developmental phase, they may not be able to start anew vocationally. They may chastise themselves for not having taken more risks or spent more time with family and friends. They too may try to make changes. Like John, they can be prone to self-destructive behavior. They often put the same intensity and energy that made them successful into these new activities. These may not always involve major changes. However, if they fail, an internal emotional vacuum is created whose symptoms can include boredom, irritability, loss of a sense of humor, moodiness, and psychosomatic concerns.(1)

Some deal with job dissatisfaction in midlife by changing jobs or even careers. Some find new challenges. Others regret it. Some keep their jobs and expand hobbies or get involved in a new avocation. Thus, they build on what they have and find new dreams. This is a viable alternative if you want to keep your job but no longer find it stimulating or cannot advance further. Learning a new skill such as carpentry, cooking, playing an instrument, scuba diving, or jogging and running in a marathon can give you new dreams and goals, keep you feeling vital, and increase your self-esteem. In any case, look before you leap. Do not quit your job until you clearly have a new job in hand.

Marriage and Other Relationships

I have seen many middle-aged men and women filled with anxiety and pain struggle in therapy as to what to do about their marital relationship. "The late forties and early fifties can be a time of agonizing reappraisal of a marital relationship, with divorce a frequent result. Although some couples survive this strain with their marriages stronger than before, even for them this time of marital transition can absorb much of their emotional energy."(2) Common areas of marital conflict involve unfulfilled needs based on unrealistic expectations, cultural differences, outside stress, communication difficulties, and unresolved childhood problems. Many themes reappear in therapy. The following are a few that may ring a bell.

A classic case is the man who brings his wife to therapy under the guise of marital counseling because he wants to soften the blow, help her adjust to the change, or keep her off his back, as he slowly leaves the relationship. The therapist is usually left to help the spouse pick up the pieces of her life and cope with the resentment engendered when she finally learns her partner's true agenda. Some come to therapy because they want to leave but are having trouble with the guilt involved in severing a long-term relationship. They say that they do not want to "hurt" the partner. The truth is that it is better to be straightforward if you really intend to leave. You can't shatter glass without there being sharp pieces. You can't avoid the anger, the pain, and the hurt. However, as soon as you tell your partner that you are leaving, he or she can start to deal with the situation and get on with life.

I have also seen cases in which the couple comes for marital counseling, but unknown to his wife, the man has a paramour, wants to stay in the marriage, and doesn't tell the spouse about the other woman. He wants to keep the status quo, and has no intention of leaving the marriage. However, he is tired of his wife's complaining about lack of attention and lack of sex. Usually he will invent an excuse not to come for therapy sessions, leaving his wife to deal with her feelings without knowing the full truth of the situation. Caught in a bind and unable to break the husband's therapeutic confidence, the therapist can usually only focus on the quality of the woman's life, help her improve her self-esteem, and encourage her to investigate new interests and hobbies. This is particularly important if it becomes apparent that the wife, although discontent in the relationship, does not want to leave.

Even sadder are the entrenched poor marriages in which neither spouse fulfills the other's needs, except perhaps for security, and both are filled with anger and defensiveness. In midlife, feeling more vulnerable and having a need for intimacy and someone to rely on, one or the other will challenge the situation. Sexual and financial issues are often used by the husband and wife to send messages to each other. The messages, if decoded, often have to do with unmet needs and desires. However, at times old resentments and hurts are too strong to allow them to figure this out. Therapy is spent ventilating years of frustration and anger, pointing fingers of blame, and leaving little energy left for constructive evaluation or change.

The Extramarital Affair

The midlife affair is often the way that some deal with internal turmoil, fear, anxiety, lost self-esteem, or a need for intimacy. It may be a way to try and deny the passage of time, rewrite the past, and/or turn back the calendar and attempt to feel young and potent again. It may be an effort to compensate for so many things. If nothing else, an affair can be interpreted as indicating that the participants are feeling needy and looking for something, perhaps attention.

In an affair, both people initially are on their best behavior and they don't have to deal with the responsibilities and daily irritations that confront married couples. For this reason, it is really unfair to compare an affair and a relationship in a marriage. It feels wonderful to be the center of attention and bask in the compliments and positive feelings that are possible in a new and limited situation. Sex may also be more satisfying as one reaches out in new ways and perhaps learns new techniques from the new partner. Sometimes the clandestine nature of the situation increases the adrenalin and adds to the adventure.

Although it may all seem good at first, will it last? What

will the relationship be like in three or four months? Will it hold up after the period of infatuation is over and some of the negative issues come to the forefront and start to give a new and realistic balance to the situation? Most important of all, what are the consequences?

Some use an affair as a transition to leave a marriage, while many return to the fold after several months. Hopefully, they have started to understand the effect an affair can have on their marital relationship, the hurt that it can bring to all concerned, and something about the true meaning of commitment. Charlotte will serve to illustrate some of these points.

Vignette: Charlotte

Charlotte was overwhelmed with anxiety and frustration when she decided to enter therapy. She had been having an affair at work for three months with a coworker. She was very dynamic and conscientious in her job. She had one teenage daughter. In her forties, she stated that everyone thought her husband was wonderful, handsome, urbane, considerate, and tolerant. Although she acknowledged that this was true, she admitted that she was obsessed with her new love and she could not get him out of her mind. She talked to him constantly at work, and was sure that she wanted to run away with him.

Charlotte was impressed with the degree of verbal intimacy she and her lover, Charles, shared. Her husband was far less verbal and tended to keep his feelings to himself. Charles constantly complained that he was in a bad marriage and disliked his wife. Charlotte said that she did not want to be the cause of his breakup, but that if he left, she also would leave her husband. In her mind, she was sure that he would leave and that they would eventually be married. In more lucid moments, she admitted that Chuck was weak and that she constantly had to make all advances and orchestrate all of their plans.

Charlotte described herself as having a strong religious and cultural family background. She revealed that as a teenager she had been shy and inhibited. Her parents had been very strict about her socialization. Her husband had been her first boyfriend, seeming much more worldly and sophisticated at the time. Having grown and matured into her own person in midlife, she suddenly found herself caught up in an emotional adventure that seemed to have a life of its own.

Coworkers began to comment on Charlotte and Chuck's relationship. She loved her job and was a valued employee. To avoid problems at work, she changed jobs, feeling that it would be easier for her to find new employment. Somehow, Charlotte's husband found out about the affair. Although visibly hurt, except for retreating to their summer home for a long weekend, he said little except that he loved her, wanted her to stop seeing Chuck, and would be supportive. Charlotte promised that she would comply, but she continued to see Chuck, who procrastinated and made excuses as to why he could not leave his wife. He spoke of his three little girls who needed him. In time, it became obvious even to Charlotte that Chuck was not going to end his marriage. Angry and frustrated, she entered therapy.

Charlotte worried about the pain she was causing her husband. She realized that although he was not as verbal or romantic as Charles, he had consistently fulfilled her needs. She admitted that their sex life had improved during her affair. He also seemed to be sharing more. She realized that she was acting like a teenager and redoing a part of her adolescence that for many reasons had been restricted the first time around. She made a firm commitment to herself not to see Chuck. This time, she kept her word. Her obsession gradually subsided.

Divorce Prevention

Therapists usually try to go with the positive in a relationship. In doing marital therapy, I will initially spend time trying to get the individuals to examine their needs and see if they can be fulfilled in the marital relationship. Sometimes after the anger is ventilated, they can look at the reasons they married their spouse in the first place. Using these good memories as a foundation, they can start to build the relationship again. At times, the patient may simply have to be taught or be given permission to ask for what they want. In both your personal life and in business, do not assume that everyone thinks the same. People cannot read your mind. People have been raised by different parents and in different emotional atmospheres. Verbalizing your needs is not a guarantee of success, but it does help. Initially in therapy, the therapist may act as the alter ego, clarifying and interpreting between the lines to help the patient better verbalize his or her feelings and needs.

Some patients seem puzzled when I talk about needs. They may say that they want their spouse to change but often cannot articulate exactly what they want them to do. Some never even conceive of themselves as having needs. We all have basic needs for food and shelter. However, we also have emotional needs for love, tenderness, intimacy, comfort, acknowledgment and acceptance, emotional support and nurturing, and affection. We also have sexual needs. Affection, for instance, is important at all ages. Some are lucky and deal with these issues instinctively and naturally. Many have difficulty here, particularly if they were deprived as a child or had parents who were not physically affectionate. They may grow up wanting physical affection but have difficulty expressing or asking for it. If encouraged, they may keep reaching out. It took a long time, and involved much trial and error, to learn to walk. The same is true for emotional gains or learning how to love.

There are other roadblocks to getting and receiving love. Anger is the most potent and the most destructive.

> It takes time to work through the initial anger and resentment that forces a couple into therapy. People must be aware of their true needs and how best to communicate them. The anger must subside before [underlying feelings of] love can be fully realized . . . Once people become aware of their need for security and companionship, feeling worthwhile and needed, and can communicate this need to their spouse, a better, more fulfilling, cooperative relationship is often possible.
>
> A relationship is an emotional equilibrium between two people. It is only when both grow that the "us" of a relationship can also grow. Both partners must maintain their individual interests,

hobbies, and concerns as well as have projects or tasks in common. The tendency for both spouses to be employed in this decade because of economic necessity or a need for self-expression has necessitated a change in the traditional roles of married people in the United States. A new equilibrium is difficult to adjust to when expectations of a traditional marriage arrangement are held. Expectations based on parental role models also can cause difficulties. Some people unconsciously expect their spouse to be like Mom or Dad.(3)

The past can influence the marital relationship in other ways. Some tend to marry people who resemble, in some of their personality characteristics, habits, or emotional tone, a parent with whom they had difficulty as a child. In a way, unconsciously, they are saying, "I didn't work it through the first time, perhaps it will come out better this time around." Sometimes, they find that they experience what I call "double trouble." The spouse tends to push the same psychological buttons as the problematic parent. The interaction would normally be upsetting. However, since it brings back memories of earlier parent–child interaction, it is doubly upsetting. For example, the woman who was raised by an alcoholic father may well find herself very emotionally troubled when dealing with the physical smell, behavior, and emotional insecurity engendered by an alcoholic spouse.

Even in a good marriage, midlife changes can cause a strain on the relationship and require some adjustment of the equilibrium. The woman who returns to the work force, takes on a career, or returns to school in midlife may have to deal with her own anxieties as well as the trials and tribulations the vocational change will have on the marital relationship. With the children out of the house and his own career established, the husband may want to spend more time with his wife at the very moment that she is immersed in her career phase and more interested in her promotion at work. The pendulum has swung. At this juncture, the man may be more interested in companionship and intimacy at a time when his wife is becoming more assertive and interested in outside work. Although he may verbalize support, resentment may rear its head as he has to spend more time alone and has to lend more of a helping hand at home.

Both partners are not always willing to come for therapy. If the partner in therapy wants the spouse to be involved, I encourage them to ask. Sometimes it is helpful and less threatening to ask them to come under the guise of being helpful to the spouse who is already there. This allows the therapist time to establish rapport and the spouse time to see that therapy is not dangerous. Sometimes one will come for one or two sessions and then find some excuse not to continue. This is particularly true of men. They often feel uncomfortable and threatened in therapy because they feel that the therapist will side with the spouse, have difficulty dealing with emotions, or don't want to put forth the effort to change. Sometimes they are wrapped so tight in their macho armor that they have difficulty acknowledging their feelings. However, there is an emotional balance between partners. "Often, even if one spouse comes for therapy, changes may soon be seen in the behavior of the other spouse."(3)

If, after careful evaluation, it is really found that the partners, having considered both the negative and positive aspects of the relationship, cannot fulfill each other's needs, it is all right to separate.

Generally, it is foolish to leave a relationship if the real problem is internal turmoil and not really the spouse or the marriage. Many men in therapy tell me that they are not any happier in a second marriage. The second wife may not have the same faults as the first, but being human, she will invariably have her own negative qualities. The second marriage may have its own set of problems, including stepchildren, increased financial responsibility, and getting used to a whole new set of personal habits and personality characteristics. The only difference the second time around seems to be that the partners are older, more willing to compromise, and work more at the relationship.

Adjusting to Postparenthood:
The Empty Nest Syndrome and Other Problems

At times, both partners do not grow equally within the framework of marriage. This can cause problems, particularly for the woman who has invested all of her energies in her growing children and has not worked outside the home. When the last child leaves home, the middle-aged woman who has been homebound and family oriented is often left with feelings of uselessness, loneliness, and depression and may develop "the empty nest syndrome." Like the man, who is left feeling this way upon retirement, it would have been helpful if she had planned ahead and developed other interests and relationships. At this juncture, she may need help to focus outside the home and reestablish relationships with her spouse and others.

Both parents must adjust to children growing up and leaving home. The empty nest syndrome is not only a feminine phenomenon. Both mothers and fathers experience emotional changes during this time. "Both parents may miss the child's company and the time he or she occupied in their lives. The parents may suddenly realize that they have missed hundreds of opportunities to have participated more actively in the child's development"(4). Fathers, particularly those who were career-oriented and not involved in child care, may experience feelings of sadness and regret that they were not closer to and more involved with the children as they were growing up. The relationship can and will continue. You will have more opportunities.

Another difficulty, during this period, is the change in how children see their parents. In the early years, they looked to them for all the answers and felt that they knew and could do everything. At times during adolescence, we get the feeling that they think we know nothing and can do nothing. But there is a light at the end of the tunnel. Usually in young adulthood, children start to see parents more realistically as human beings with both good and bad points. The relationship becomes one between two adults rather than just parent and child.

> The parent–child relationship is unique.... Both adolescents and their parents have a multitude of memories of common experiences. Parents have nurtured their children and watched them develop and in this process have acquired a kind of attachment that is significantly different from any other.... Parents have mixed feelings about their children becoming mature. Although tending to be proud of their developing adolescents, they may at the same time be reluctant to lose them as children.(2)

It is difficult to disengage and let go of your children. Parents who are too devoted or overprotective may slow down or hinder the adolescent's move toward independence. As we stressed in Chapter 4, let them go. They will return. A new equilibrium will be established and the relationship will continue. Don't clutch onto your children. The relationship must change. Fifty percent of the outcome is under your control; the other half is up to the adolescent. Some parents who have difficulty with change cause themselves much pain by holding on too tight. It is important for adolescents to realize that in seeking independence, they need to allow time for parents to adjust. Be kind to one another. Don't close the door on your relationship. Keep trying. One day, you may look back and wonder what all the heat was about.

The empty nest or postparenthood phase of life does not have to be depressing. Some studies have shown that it indeed can be a good time of life.(5) The children leaving home may usher in a new and positive stage of life for parents. Relieved of the restrictions of childrearing, they can spend more time establishing new interests, investing in others, and working on marital satisfaction. It can be a second honeymoon period. As we shall see, contact with aging parents, continued contact with growing children, and the advent of grandparenthood will soon fill any gap, making you feel quite needed and emotionally gratified once again.

Middle-Age Stress

"A difficult situation, even for normal-average people, has the potential for producing a stress reaction. Coping mechanisms fail when something in your world causes a threat to life, a risk of injury, or a loss of security. Change and adjustment are part of life. Therefore, the stress of life can affect us all."(6) This is particularly true during midlife when we are faced with a complex of changes and challenges.

Living with stress can produce symptoms of anxiety, including feelings of restlessness, heart palpitations, irritability, and tension. It can produce somatic complaints such as headaches and muscular aches and pains. Behavioral disturbances can occur, such as increased smoking, drug and alcohol abuse, and compulsive gambling. Marital problems, outbursts of temper, and overreaction to minor issues will be seen. Depression as a reaction to loss can show itself through withdrawal, poor appetite, and sleep disturbances.

Stress can also contribute to physical illness. Hypertension, asthma, migraine headaches, heart disease, allergies, ulcer disease, and irritable bowel syndrome often have an emotional component linked to stress. Stress can be associated with failure to menstruate and impotence. Stress weakens the body's defense mechanisms and reduces its resistance to infection. There may even be a link between emotional stress and cancer.

There are three basic alternatives to any stress situation:

1. Do something to change the situation.
2. Get out of it.
3. Change yourself so as to live more comfortably with it.

More specifically, here are some things you can do to reduce stress in midlife.

Improve communication skills. Good communication is a buffer against increased stress. It is an important asset in both business and marital relationships. Good communication includes such techniques as looking at your own and other's feelings, really listening attentively to others, giving feedback, expressing your wishes more effectively, and checking out your assumptions. We can't just assume that our expectations and assumptions are universal. Ask directly for what you want. It is not a guarantee of success, but people cannot read your mind.

In therapy, I often make use of the ideas of transactional analysis to help patients improve their interactions. This is a school of psychotherapy developed by Eric Berne(7), who felt that emotional problems developed and are maintained in the context of relationships. For Berne, each of us has a set of feelings, thoughts, and behavior patterns related to a child, adult, and parent ego state. We communicate in these states at various times in relationships and can elicit child, adult, or parental responses from others. These characteristic ways of relating can be changed. He talks about how we relate to people in various "transactions," including that of parent/child and more effectively as adult/adult. This can be a helpful reference point in understanding what is going on in certain communications between people.

Talk to someone. Talk out your problems and share your feelings. The support of your friends and family is crucial. Ask for reassurance and even physical contact if you need it. Women in general are more apt to ask for help and are more comfortable talking about feelings. Men on the other hand tend to deal more with facts. "The ancient myth that men must be strong, potent, unflappable, that any sign of emotion signals weakness or passivity, had done the male species more harm than good over the years. Because men have a hard time expressing their inner feelings . . . the resulting phenomenon is a feeling of isolation which brings on stress that is manifested in many different forms."(8)

Release your tension. Find ways to work off your feelings of frustration and excess aggressive energy. Exercise works for many. It's never too late to start. Regular exercise, sports, or even walking can counter and dispel the tension associated with stress. Combating isolation by getting involved with others in community, religious, and philanthropic groups is helpful for some and can give you a perspective. Relaxation techniques can be easily learned.

Have realistic expectations. Unrealistic expectations are a leading cause of stress. Burnout occurs when unrealistically high expectations cause you to experience emotional and physical fatigue. "Your expectations in a situation are important. It is not really the external situation that causes stress but rather the way that a person deals with the problem. People who value control over sharing their feelings are more likely to show signs of stress. . . . Those who recognize and accept their own limitations and take a problem-solving approach to life will do better."(6)

Learn to manage time efficiently. Time pressure is another leading cause of stress. Trouble arises when you try to take on too much responsibility or expect to accomplish everything. The main stress inducer is having too much to do and too little control over the time and manner in which it is done. This will be particularly important to remember if you are in the work force, dealing with children and adolescents, coordinating a household, or being a caregiver to the elderly. Often conscientious people follow the maxim that if they do everything right, everything will work out all right. This can often cause disappointment and frustration. It is important to establish boundaries between your various roles and to set limits for the use of your time.

Use professional help. A full range of mental health services is available in most communities. Mental health groups such as Recovery, Inc., let you know that you are not alone or unique and provide support for many. National, state, and local organizations can be used as a resource to obtain information on specific disorders and sources of professional help. Don't be afraid or ashamed to ask. You are probably not losing control or going crazy. Even normal-average people react to stress. There are things to do to help yourself. If these do not seem to work or if your reaction is prolonged and interfering with your life, ask for help.

All human beings are prone to stress. However, what is stressful to one may not be stressful to another. Although we all go through a midlife transition, some suffer more and are more upset by the process. What makes the difference? "My guess is that it has a lot to do with expectations, with the willingness to verbalize concerns, with the availability of support systems, with role models. . . . And with luck. We have to have enough luck at the right time."(9) Other issues that make a difference are being comfortable with yourself, knowing how to ask for help, and realizing that there is more to life than just work. Enjoy yourself and your family.(10)

Guidelines for Success

- Look before you leap in making job, career, or marital changes.
- Do not quit your job until you clearly have another in hand.
- Change is not always the answer, particularly if the problem is internal turmoil. Talk it out with an objective person.
- Don't throw it all away. Build on what you have.
- Reevaluate your expectations and goals more realistically. Formulate a new dream.
- Do not close the door on relationships. Tomorrow is another day.
- An assertive problem-solving approach is best.
- Verbalize your feelings and concerns.
- Ask for what you want.
- Take a risk and do something new.
- It's all right to slow down a little and take care of yourself. Know your limits.

- Decrease isolation and increase support systems.
- Pay attention to the quality of your life.
- Make peace with who you are.
- Be optimistic.
- Hope for a little bit of luck.

Chapter 9

The Middle-Aged Mind and Body

Shattered Dreams and Expectations

Middle age can present unsettling new realities. Psychologically, it is a time for letting go of illusions and dealing with the disappointment of unrealized ambitions, especially the grandiose expectations of adolescence and young adulthood. It is a time to update and perhaps remodel life's goals. It is also a time to come to terms with and accept the limitations of one's self and of one's loved ones. Added to these emotional changes are the more concrete physical changes that occur as bodily health, long taken for granted, becomes less dependable and predictable and illness comes more and more out of the shadows. "In this phase, a new anxiety is added . . . the anxiety of loss of function, decay, and death."(1)

> The issues of waning strength, fading beauty, biological clocks, the aging and death of parents, the departure from home of adolescent children, lost opportunities and renunciation of aspirations, and perhaps most important, the erosion of one's denial that life is finite and death inevitable are indeed the stressful challenges of the middle years.(2)

Add to all this worries about the prospects of retirement or the increasing loneliness of those who never married or are divorced or widowed, and you start to gain a picture of the impact of this time period on the middle-aged mind and body. Just as midlife can be about challenge, exploring new vistas, creative living, and generativity, it is also about shattered dreams and expectations. Change and fear of the unknown can lead to anxiety; loss can lead to mourning and depression. This negative side of midlife if prolonged can serve as a detour away from maturity and contentment.

In therapy, Nora (see Chapter 1) had some understanding of this process. She often posed questions such as "When will I be myself again? When will my husband be himself again? When is this woman going to get well and be my mother again?" Symbolically, these questions signified the changes that were occurring in Nora's life, and the losses she was sustaining. Even as she tried desperately to work through her midlife emotional distress and accept the multiple changes occurring in her self and her world, she continued to long for the past and its predictable comforts. None of these people, including Nora, would ever be the same again. They would never be young again.

Midlife Depression

Midlife can manifest any psychiatric symptoms or syndromes. Hormone imbalance, menopause, and the "midlife crisis" can not be blamed for all midlife emotional disturbances. A full range of diagnoses, including neuroses, personality disorders, and psychoses, is possible. Regression to schizophrenia or manic depressive illness may occur under the stress of important events in the life cycle, particularly in those with a past history of these disorders. However, one of the most common emotional sequelae during this period is depression. It can result from the real and imagined physical and emotional losses and changes and diminished self-esteem that can occur in both sexes during this time.

Life's normal progression during middle age can create situations that precipitate feelings of sadness, mourning, and depression. We all have experienced the "blahs" or a passing "blue" mood, but clinical depression is different. Psychologically, depression can be seen as a reaction to a specific loss or change, such as the children leaving home, or due to some life experience or stress that ordinarily produces sadness, such as a death in the family, business reverses, financial losses, and rejection. Midlife brings additional outside pressures that can precipitate mood changes. Parents grow older and are often sick. Careers and relationships may not be as satisfying.

Diagnostically, these types of depression care are called *dysthymia* (depressive neurosis) or *major depression*. Dysthymia is a mild depression that is chronic, lasting at least two years. In addition to a depressed mood, the patient must show at least two of the other clinical symptoms listed below. In a major depression, the patient has a depressed mood that lasts longer than two weeks and shows at least five of the symptoms listed below. In these types of depression, the reaction is appropriate but prolonged.

The traditional adult clinical picture of depression can include the following symptoms:

1. A persistent depressed, down, sad, empty, or blue mood.
2. Loss of enjoyment or interest in usual activities including sex.
3. Decreased energy, fatigue, feeling slowed down and tired.
4. Sleep problems, including difficulty falling asleep, staying asleep, early morning awakening, or sleeping too much.
5. Poor appetite, weight loss, or overeating.
6. Feeling worthless, guilty, helpless, or blaming one's self for things.
7. Feeling hopeless, pessimistic, or wondering if life is worth living.
8. Difficulty in concentration, memory, and making decisions.
9. Worrying or stewing about things.

10. Feeling irritable, agitated, restless, and anxious.
11. Persistent crying spells.
12. Chronic aches and pains and other physical problems that don't seem to respond to treatment.
13. Recurrent thoughts of death or suicide.

Depression occurring for the first time in middle age or beyond in men or women can be more severe and involve changes in the person's ability to test reality. These depressions are considered to be of psychotic proportions. Major affective disorder with psychotic features was previously called a psychotic depressive reaction. Many years ago, it was called an involutional psychotic reaction ("involutional" referring to the biological retrograde or degenerative changes that occur between ages 40 to 65). Regardless of which name is used, this type of depression is also a reactive depression attributable to some experience. Here the clinical characteristics described previously are seen but in a more intense and severe form. In addition, there is impairment in reality testing. Delusions (false beliefs) are present usually involving depressive themes such as disease, punishment, death, or personal inadequacy. Hallucinations can be present, and the patient's ability to function is impaired.

Major depression may also be of melancholic type, which corresponds to the older diagnosis of involutional melancholia. Here there is a gradual onset of severe depression which occurs in the involutional period. There is usually an absence of prior episodes. This illness occurs particularly in those who have a rigid and compulsive premorbid personality. This reaction is manifested by intractable insomnia, suicidal ruminations, worry, anxiety, and much guilt. Marked changes in bodily functions, including severe anorexia, weight loss, and constipation, occur. There can be psychomotor retardation or agitation.

The involutional period can also bring about an involutional paranoid state or what is now called a delusional (paranoid) disorder. Here the delusions or false beliefs are not due to any other mental disorder. They involve real-life situations rather than bizarre ideas or events. Patients with this disorder may complain that they are being followed or mistreated, have a serious disease, are loved by an important person, or are being deceived by their sexual partner. Auditory or visual hallucinations are not prominent.

Substance Abuse and Other Crutches

As we have noted, the changes and challenges of the middle years can be stressful. During this time, middle-aged men and women may deny, minimize, or cover up their internal turmoil and then drink, use other substances, or other self-defeating crutches to deal with their tensions. The following vignette shows how such behavior can reflect psychological stress, as we watch Jenny try to cope with her multiple responsibilities.

Vignette: Jenny

Jenny lost her job last year due to a change in administration. She was quite frustrated and angry. She has been unable to find new employment. Her mother has been very sick and Jenny has had to care for her in her home. Recently, Jenny has been very irritable and fighting frequently with her husband, particularly over how to raise their three [teenage] children.

She always had one or two drinks at night after work to relax. During the last six months, the number of drinks had started to increase and she had started to gulp them. Recently, Jenny started drinking in the morning to help her get through the day. Her family grew concerned and spoke to her. She blamed her marital problems for her drinking and maintained that she didn't have a problem.

She started to let her housework go and found that she occasionally woke up and didn't remember what had happened to her. On June 30, she fell down the stairs and had to be admitted to the hospital with a broken wrist.

It finally hit home, Jenny could no longer deny her problem. She felt as if she were losing control. She picked up the phone and dialed the number her family physician had given her in order to enter the 28-day inpatient alcoholic treatment program. At last, she was reaching out for help.(3)

Jenny is not alone. Many people in middle age escalate bad habits such as overeating, smoking, or the recreational use of illegal drugs or alcohol to deal with the stresses of midlife. Other crutches can include excessive gambling, the overuse of legal drugs such as sedative-hypnotics, or sexual acting out through an extramarital affair. Some will get into difficulty taking tranquilizers or antidepressants belonging to friends or other family members, without professional evaluation. Even average citizens, following the false dictum of the popular media image of a pill for every need, can fall into this trap.

As in Jenny's case, this behavior often reflects psychological stress. She was dealing with the loss of her job, the new responsibilities brought on by her mother's illness, and her family problems. Escalating her intake of alcohol was the maladaptive way she dealt with her feelings of depression and anger. Alcoholism is a disease involving the body, mind, and spirit. But, as with Jenny, it is also a sign that a person is trying to cope with problems of life. It is a sign that there are underlying emotional problems and serious unmet needs.

Sexual Issues

Midlife can enhance or inhibit sexuality for both men and women. The quality and enjoyment of sex does not have to change in midlife. If anything, reduced anxiety and increased knowledge of a partner's body and their likes and dislikes can increase the pleasure. Age does bring some modification of sexual responsiveness. Men will achieve erection more slowly and women will have a decrease in the number of orgasmic contractions. More foreplay may be necessary to stimulate arousal. Men may be more easily distracted and require a more peaceful sexual environment. Menopausal women may develop atrophic vaginitis and require hormonal replacement and/or extra lubrication.

For many women, having their menses is an important confirmation of womanhood and normalcy. They often tie their sexual activity strictly to their procreative function and they no longer feel entitled to enjoy sexual activity when they are unable to reproduce. Many women are relieved not to menstruate when they know that menopause is a normal life event and that there is nothing wrong with them or their bodies. Some will be relieved not to have to use birth control, which may have been an impediment to the full expression of their sexuality, and a health worry due to reports of breast cancer, heart disease, and phlebitis. They may have a renaissance of libido at this time due to decreased female hormones leaving the endogenic influence unopposed.

The lack of male potency and sex drive has many causes. These include psychological factors such as boredom, depression, and stress. Male erectile dysfunction can also be related to health status such as fatigue, vascular and hormonal disorders, alcohol and drug abuse, and nutritional deficiencies. It can also be affected by medication, such as antihypertensive drugs, and physical disorders, such as diabetes mellitus.

A menopausal wife can have an affect on some men. Such men feel that they no longer have to perform for a wife who is biologically unable to bear children. Religious beliefs may also play a role. However, these men often have been looking for an excuse to terminate sexual activity with their spouses. On the other hand, men who have been inconvenienced by the need for birth control now may feel terrific because they can enjoy unimpeded sexual activity. The psychological effect of aging can also affect sexual attitudes in the male. The middle-aged male may cast aside his aging spouse because she reminds him that he is also aging.(4) Psychoanalytically, some speculate that an aging wife may remind the husband of his mother, the forbidden love object. Unable to deal with this psychological stress, he may turn to a younger partner.(5)

Having a growing, particularly midadolescent, teenager in the house may also affect parental feelings about their own bodies and their own sexuality. This, of course, will depend on the parents' degree of emotional maturity. For some, comparisons may cause feelings of sexual inadequacy, envy, and competition rather than pleasure and pride. Seeing your child grow into a physically robust individual who suddenly has the ability to be sexually stimulating and provocative can also make you more aware of your own age and the fact that you will never be sixteen again. This can lead to feelings of loss and depression. "The adolescent's blossoming sexuality may stir up the middle-aged parent's earlier unresolved conflicts around sexuality—envy, competition, fear, guilt—may lead to guilty and competitive prohibitions, fascinated encouragement, and acting out on everybody's part."(6)

Health Worries

Many middle-aged people seem to worry about their health. This is a common concern I hear in therapy. It is a frequent cause of anxiety in this age group. Many who have been in good health until midlife find it difficult to deal with the unpredictable physical changes of this time of life relinquish the myth that they are invincible, and accept new limitations.

As an intern working in the emergency room, I quickly learned to put physical symptoms in perspective. For instance, every person who came in with a bad cough was not presumed to have tuberculosis or lung cancer. They may simply have a bad cold or upper respiratory infection. We were taught to rule out simple illnesses first and then move up the ladder of differential diagnoses. This is good to keep in mind when evaluating your own physical symptoms. Anxious people particularly seem to anticipate the worst in a situation, immediately assuming that they are seriously ill or that they may die. The above approach is one way to keep from catastrophizing, which can only increase anxiety and total discomfort.

Having a growing, vibrantly healthy adolescent in the house may also further complicate the situation of the middle-aged individual with waning physical powers and vigor. Comparisons can stimulate the same kind of feelings of physical envy, inadequacy, competition, and/or loss that we saw in the sexual sphere. Feelings about your health can also be influenced by the physical and mental health and vitality of your aging parents. Their decline can often cause you anxiety about your own physical position and force you to confront your own vulnerability and mortality. Serious illness and physical disability suffered by a parent may also stimulate tension and doubts about your own present and future health.

Questions about your physical and mental health are best left to your own physician to answer. He or she knows you and your medical and family history and can best diagnose and treat you. I offer the following information about some of the medical problems that can start in middle age, as well as guidelines for good physical health in midlife, only to increase your awareness and give you a perspective. This information is not intended as a substitute for professional medical care. If you think you see yourself in the following descriptions, please make an appointment with your doctor for further evaluation, reassurance, and an individualized treatment plan.

Seeing your doctor, checking out your assumptions, and having a correct diagnosis can do much to reduce your anxiety about your health. Some still avoid going for evaluation or overreact emotionally to being told that they have something physically wrong. This may be due to a fear of the unknown, lack of accurate information, or distorted memories of a parent or relative with a similar disorder. After you have checked out the facts, try to remember that your health, although very important, is only one aspect of your life. Don't overreact and see everything as black. Think about how content and happy you are in the other spheres of your life such as your work, family, friends, community involvement, and hobbies. Don't let your distress spoil it all. Follow your doctor's medical advice, but continue to enjoy your joys and pleasures. Allow your happy moments to help you accept your health situation and put the medical problem in perspective.

The following are some of the physical disorders that can first appear and be diagnosed in midlife.

Cardiovascular

Hypertension
Hypercholesterolemia/hyperlipidemia
Coronary artery disease

Respiratory

Chronic obstructive pulmonary disease

Gastrointestinal

Bowel cancer
Gall bladder disease
Peptic ulcer disease

Musculoskeletal

Back pain
Degenerative joint disease/osteoarthritis
Osteoporosis

Endocrine

Menopause
Adult onset diabetes
Hypothyroidism
Breast cancer

Genito-urinary

Benign prostatic hyperplasia (BPH)
Stress incontinence

Neurological

Presbyopia (long sight and impairment of vision)
Presbycusis (diminished acuteness of hearing)

Hypertension. Hypertension or high blood pressure has been called a "silent disease" because it has no characteristic symptoms until it reaches an advanced state. It is present when the blood pressure exceeds 140/90 mm Hg. You may become aware of it only in a routine blood pressure reading or physical exam. A few people may receive a clue to its presence through symptoms such as headaches, tiredness, dizziness, or nosebleeds. Treatment is important. Take your medication prescribed. Untreated, it can lead to serious complications such as coronary artery disease, congestive heart failure, stroke, and kidney damage.

Although sixty million Americans have hypertension, the cause of the disease is usually unknown. Such cases are called "primary or essential" hypertension. Secondary hypertension, although less common, has an identifiable cause such as kidney disease or a hormonal imbalance. Several factors seem to increase the risk of developing hypertension, including a family history, being a female over fifty, being black, smoking, heavy alcohol consumption, obesity, dietary salt, and stress.(7, 8)

Hypercholesterolemia. Cholesterol is a yellow, waxy molecule produced by the liver whose job it is to carry digested fat to parts of the body where it is used for energy and repairs or to fat storage sties such as the hips or abdomen. The liver makes up packages called lipoproteins, which consist of lipids (fat and cholesterol) and protein. There are three types of lipoproteins: very low-density lipoprotein (VLDL), low-density lipoprotein (LDL), and high-density lipoprotein (HDL). VLDL (mostly triglycerides) becomes LDL (low-density lipoprotein) after it unloads fat. LDL is called "bad" cholesterol because it easily becomes stuck along blood vessel walls as it is returning to the liver. Knowing your LDL level is important. It can help you put the cholesterol story into perspective. It should be less than 160.

$$LDL = \text{Total cholesterol} - \frac{\text{Triglycerides}}{5} - HDL$$

HDL is called "good" cholesterol. It finds and removes stuck LDL and brings it back to the liver to be either recycled or excreted. HDL under 35 is a risk factor for coronary heart disease.

$$\text{Total cholesterol} = \text{HDL} + \text{LDL} + \text{VLDL}$$

Your total cholesterol should be less than 200. If you eat too much fat, the entire transport process increases. Blood vessels can become narrowed or blocked, causing problems such as a heart attack, peripheral vascular disease, or stroke. There are five subtypes of hypercholesterolemia: I, IIa, IIb, III, IV, and V. Some are inherited, some can be controlled by diet alone, and some must be treated with diet and medication. We cannot control risk factors for coronary heart disease such as family history of premature heart disease or being male. However, we can control risk factors such as high cholesterol, high blood pressure, smoking, and obesity.

Back Pain. Back pain can be excruciating. Pain in the lower back or lumbo-sacral region of the spinal column usually occurs spontaneously. It can signal an injury, structural or neurological changes, a herniated (ruptured) disc, arthritis, or a tumor. However, most commonly, the pain is caused by weakness of the muscles around the spine, an abnormal position, or posture which puts pressure on or "pinches" a nerve as it passes through the openings between the vertebrae. Pain can also occur when muscles that have been misused or are not used to exercise go into spasm. Chronic problems in this area can cause people to limit their activity because they fear precipitating pain, reinjuring themselves, or are experiencing secondary gain.

Osteoarthritis. Osteoarthritis is the most common of the more than 100 forms of arthritis. It is also called degenerative joint disease (DJD). An age-related deterioration of articular cartilage and underlying bone, it is often described as "wear-and-tear" disease. Osteoarthritis initiates metabolic changes that cause joint cartilage to degenerate. Here the cartilage, the cushion or smooth lining covering the ends of bones in joints so they don't grate against each other, gradually breaks down or wears thin. As a consequence, the bones begin to rub against each other and spurs and nodes can form. Deformity can occur late in the disease.

Osteoarthritis usually only affects one or two areas, most commonly the fingers, spine, hips, and knees. Signs and symptoms of osteoarthritis vary with the joint involved and the severity of the disease. Joint aches and pain start to occur with movement. Muscle weakness may result if you avoid using the joint due to discomfort. Other complaints include stiffness, most noticeable upon arising (morning stiffness) or during damp, cold weather. Renewed stiffness can occur after prolonged inactivity. Swelling, inflammation, warmth, and tenderness can occur. A grinding sound can sometimes be heard when a joint is put through a full range of motion.(9)

Menopause. As we stated in Chapter 7, menopause is a natural physiological life event and not an illness. It is a normal process which represents the cessation of the menstrual cycle and the end of the childbearing years. It usually occurs in American women between the ages of 48 and 55. You may know that menopause is starting when you experience changes in your menstrual cycle, such as decreased bleeding, skipped or irregular periods, or heavy bleeding. The process may take six months to two years.

Many of the physical changes associated with menopause are caused by a change in hormonal balance, particularly estrogen loss.(10,11) These include:

1. Hot flashes.
2. Thinning of the vaginal lining.
3. Pelvic relaxation symptoms such as cystocele, rectocele, and stress incontinence.
4. Vaginal itching and dryness.
5. Skin changes (thinning and drying).
6. Change in breast firmness and shape due to diminished glandular tissue.

7. Hair changes—thinning and possible increase in facial and body hair.
8. Osteoporosis.
9. Weight gain (this may really be due to decrease in activity without any decrease in food intake).

Adult Onset Diabetes. Adult onset diabetes, also called non-insulin-dependent diabetes mellitus (NIDDM) or Type II diabetes, is the most common form of diabetes. Genetics and obesity are factors in causation. Here insulin is produced, but the pancreas is "lazy" and produces less insulin secretion, or the body is resistant and does not respond as well to the effect of insulin. The pancreas may need external stimulation in the form of medication to wake it up or shake it to produce insulin. Symptoms that would alert one to possible insulin deficiency or high blood sugar include increased thirst, urination, and appetite. There can also be weight loss, weakness, and fatigue. Diabetes can also cause blurred vision, skin infections, and numbness or tingling of the toes and fingers.

Stress incontinence. This is the involuntary discharge of urine due to straining, coughing, sneezing or laughing, or anything else that causes pressure in the pelvic area. It is caused by the stretching of the pelvic muscles and fibrous tissues caused by pregnancy as well as the physical changes of aging. These include relaxation of the muscles in the pelvis which cause the angle of the bladder to change, relaxation of the sphincter (outlet) muscles of the bladder, and hormonal changes which cause atrophy or thinning of the tissues in the area.

The Middle-Age Health Exam

A yearly physical exam is recommended for all those over age 40. The following is a general outline of the physical exam that your physician may do. Particular emphasis is placed on preventive medicine. With a middle-aged patient, the physician will have to keep in mind certain high-risk groups, such as those with a family history of diabetes; persons with multiple sexual partners; those whose occupation or travel history brought them in contact with certain diseases; cardiac risk factors; a family history of cancer; and perimenopausal women with increased risk to osteoporosis. He will also have to keep in mind the leading causes of death in middle age, including heart disease, lung cancer, cerebrovascular disease, breast cancer, colorectal cancer, and obstructive lung disease. He will have to remain alert for depressive symptoms, suicide risk factors, abnormal bereavement, signs of physical abuse or neglect, malignant skin lesions, peripheral arterial disease, tooth decay, gingivitis, and loose teeth.(12)

History

Diet/appetite/weight loss or gain

Physical activity

Tobacco/alcohol/drug use

Sexual practices

Review of recent medications

Allergies

Past medical problems such as scarlet fever, rheumatic fever, jaundice, malaria, TB, anemia, seizures, asthma, malignancies, typhoid fever, or arthritis

Recent trips or vacations, particularly out of the country

Prior surgeries or hospitalizations

History of having had a transfusion and when

Family history of physical problems such as hypertension, diabetes, kidney stones, gout, arthritis, heart disease, allergies, bleeding problems or cancer

Family and/or personal history of emotional problems and/or treatment

Systems Review: This will include skin, head, eyes, ears, nose, throat, neck, respiratory, cardiovascular, gastrointestinal, genito-urinary, ob/gyn, endocrine musculoskeletal, and neuropsychiatric, with particular attention to the following:

Intolerance of weather changes

History of unusual skin lesions, rashes, excessive bruising

History of blurred vision, ringing in the ears, nose bleeds, or frequent upper respiratory infections

History of chest pain, shortness of breath (when getting up at night), tiring easily with activity, severe headaches, numbness of fingers, or swelling of ankles and legs

Increased thirst or urination, dry or oily skin, unusual activity level (overactive or fatigued)

Pain when urinating, urinary frequency or urgency, difficulty starting urinating, and strength of stream (in men)

Diarrhea or constipation

Stiffness or redness of the joints

Menstrual history, including any recent changes (female)

Pain or discomfort in testicles (male)

Physical Examination

Height and weight

Blood pressure

General head to toe physical exam including:

Complete skin exam

Eye exam

Oral cavity exam

Palpation of thyroid

Auscultation of carotid bruits

Clinical breast exam for both men and women (yearly for women)

Rectal exam including prostate palpation in males

Pelvic exam (female)

Flexible sigmoidoscopy (beginning at age 50 for both men and women)

Laboratory Tests/Diagnostic Procedures

Electrocardiogram (EKG)

Mammogram (baseline age 35, particularly for those at increased risk; every 2 years until age 50; and then every year)
Papanicolaou Smear (Pap Test)
Complete blood count (CBC)
Urinalysis
Cholesterol profile
Fecal occult blood
Hearing test
High risk groups:

  Pulmonary function test
  Fasting plasma glucose
  VDRL/RPR
  Chlamydeal testing
  Gonorrhea culture
  Counseling and testing for HIV
  Tuberculin skin test
  Bone mineral content

Guidelines for Success

A friend once joked to me that middle age is the time of life when our bodies fall apart. This is certainly not literally true, although physical changes do occur. Midlife is a time that requires better maintenance than was necessary in the earlier years. It may be important to make certain life-style changes. I therefore offer the following guidelines for good physical health in midlife. These points are only meant to start you thinking. See your own physician for clarification, further information, and individualized advice.

- *Follow good rules of nutrition.* As your body grows older, your need for nutrition increases and your need for calories decreases. We tend to absorb some nutrients somewhat less efficiently as we age. Therefore, focus on nutrient-dense foods which are loaded with vitamins, minerals, and fiber but are low in fat and calories. They include dark green and orange vegetables, fruits, whole-grain cereals and breads, beans and peas, and low-fat dairy products. A healthful middle-age diet plan should also be calcium rich, high in fish, emphasize complex carbohydrates (pasta, rice, barley, and potatoes), and avoid fried foods.

- *Halt the salt.* Do not put salt on your food and avoid sodium-rich foods such as potato chips, pickles, and some prepared foods. Salt has been linked to hypertension and fluid retention.
- *Reduce or eliminate caffeine.* Remember that tea as well as many soft drinks contain caffeine.
- *Stop smoking.* Cigarette smoking is a controllable risk factor for heart and pulmonary disease.
- *Lose extra pounds.* Overweight can be a factor in diabetes and cardiovascular and hypertensive disease, as well as in problems with mobility, such as arthritis and gout. It can also be a factor in back pain and other musculoskeletal disorders. There is no easy solution. Weight loss can only be achieved when you take in less food and do more exercise.
- *Avoid empty calories.* These are found in alcohol, rich desserts, and candy.
- *Exercise.* Establish and stick to a sensible exercise program for optimum body functioning. Exercise stimulates circulation and helps maintain muscle tone, agility, and stamina. Exercise is also an excellent way to reduce tension. Build up your exercise routine gradually and avoid overexertion.
- *Vitamins.* A vitamin and mineral supplement may be helpful. Your needs are best determined by your doctor.
- *Get sufficient rest.* Sleep deprivation can build up over time.
- *Relax.* Eat in a pleasant and unhurried atmosphere. Leave time in your busy schedule to unwind and to do some of the things you want to do.

- *Have a yearly physical examination.* It is also good practice to see your doctor when you first notice a change in your body or general health.
- *Take good care of yourself.* If you don't, who will?

Life is often a struggle. As you have seen in the last three chapters, middle age can be a challenge requiring a reassessment of your body, mind, and environment. Regardless of the presenting complaint, a certain acceptance of the human condition is necessary to make progress. People must be accepted as human; expectations must be realistic; perfection must be seen as wishful thinking; and reality must replace fantasy. You must push forward in a problem-solving manner to be successful in business or in life. The stages of life are full of trials and tribulations that teach valuable lessons. Middle age is no different. With a little insight, the correction of some misconceptions, and an ability to laugh at yourself, you can overcome some of the hurdles and find that life also can be fulfilling and good.(13)

Perhaps part of the answer is not to expect life to always be the same. In midlife, we need to accept a new physical vulnerability, take care of ourselves, count our blessings, and strive for contentment. Nora (see Chapter 1), like all of us, soon realized that there were some things she could not control. She had lost a little in the physical sphere but had gained immensely in the area of wisdom, confidence, self-esteem, and interpersonal relationships. She gradually accepted the changes in herself and the ones she loved. She laughed when this realization finally fell into place for her. One day in therapy she said, "Perhaps this new gang I'm going around with is OK."

Just as you have said goodbye to the kids, gotten used to their being out of the house, and started to accept your new middle-aged self, new events may occur that further complicate your life and test your emotional and physical strength. Suddenly, your aging parent(s), the other side of the midlife sandwich, may be retiring and/or require additional attention due to illness or disability. Just as you start to relax and take some time for yourself, you may be required to reverse the parent–child role and become a caregiver to your mother, father, in-law, or other aging relative. Let's look at the issues involved in this transition.

Chapter 10

Middle-Aged Children and Their Aging Parents

The parent–child bond continues to change in midlife as middle-aged children deal with their aging parents. In this process, the middle-aged individual establishes a new emotional equilibrium. According to psychoanalytic theory(1), an internal psychic change occurs during adolescence as we separate or individuate from our parents, form our own identity, and establish autonomy. As we have seen, many of the adolescent's actions clearly say, "This is me!" This process is similar to the one that occurs toward the end of the second year of life, when the child differentiates between itself and others by emphatically stating, "No!"

It has been suggested that another interpsychic change takes place in middle age due to the aging and death of one's parents.(2) Although this "third individuation" can lead to a more mature sense of self, it can be a stressful process, bringing about depression and regression. It can be one more cause of the "midlife crisis" as it reactivates old unresolved conflicts, creates anxiety, and at times precipitates adolescent-like problematic behavior.

Standing Alone

Part of the turmoil of midlife is the realization at some point that you are alone. There is no one inside you but yourself.

Although those in your life may love you and be supportive, you are responsible for your own actions and decisions. Growing up and joining the adult world means independence, responsibility, and commitment. This realization can often be precipitated by the death of a parent or others of their generation on whom you psychologically leaned for support in time of crisis. In any case, the parental aging process, as it gradually transforms you into the caregiver, soon makes you aware that you must stand on your own and that you can no longer always rely on parents for strength, comfort, and help.

Many struggle with these issues in psychotherapy. At first, it can be scary to grapple with the concept of independence. Working toward being a mature adult can be anxiety-producing. The end-result can be a heightened sense of security and pride in your abilities. Some must learn that they are capable of standing alone psychologically. Others find that they have really been self-sufficient for a long time but always thought, "If I need them [parents], they are there." Therefore, they feel psychologically unbalanced when the person they felt they could depend on in a crisis is no longer available.

Patients are often not aware of their dependency needs or how they handle these needs psychologically. Many people transfer the image of a strong parent on whom they can rely to a spouse whom they see as capable, reliable, and strong. Conversely, they often picture themselves as weak although they may be quite competent. In my work, for instance, with panic disorder patients, I have seen this as an issue. Loss or threat of loss of a significant other can remove a psychological anchor and serve as an emotional etiological factor in precipitating panic disorder.(3)

Role Reversal

We tend to take our parents' good health and existence for granted. We wear emotional blinders and assume that they will always be healthy, viable, and there to fulfill our needs. At some point in middle age a subtle transition or shift occurs in the parent–child relationship. Suddenly, out of the blue, you realize that Mom and Dad have aged. You may be walking behind them down the street or glance at them across the room. You really look at them and realize that they are walking a little slower, have a little less zest, and are a lot grayer than you remembered. The insight may come after they have suffered an illness or an accident. In any case, the moment comes when it dawns on you that they are vulnerable, human, and not invincible. You realize that they are getting old. Nothing does more to mellow old hurts, help resolve old issues, and start to work toward a new relationship based on acceptance and appreciation.

More slowly, another shift takes place. As the train of life moves on, your parents begin to show additional signs of physical and mental wear and tear. You find that you need and want to be there to fulfill their needs. You begin to take on the role of caregiver. You watch them deal with retirement, react to the loss of old friends and loved ones, and at some point even struggle with the idea of nursing-home placement. Death may come to one or the other, leaving you with your own grief. But all the while you have to be there to help them live again after the loss of a spouse. At each new station, their pain is your pain, and you struggle to help them cope.

These changes can be seen as a loss and produce a mourning process. Judith Viorst, author of the book *Necessary Losses,* sums it up well.

> We may mourn the realization that there are many things we no longer can get from our parents, many things that we never got, and never will. We may mourn the end of our dream of forever and ever being our parents' protected child. We may mourn the difficult fact that, with the reversal of parent–child roles—whether we're ready or not—it's grown-up time now. And watching our once-so-powerful parents marked by the passage of time, we may mourn the mother and father who "used to be."(4)

Resolving Old Issues

The parent–child relationship is a frequent topic for discussion in therapy. Many patients carry a lot of old baggage or old business from the past with them into middle age. This is particularly true today, when our professional jargon includes such concepts as the dysfunctional family, and we are acutely aware of "the child within" à la John Bradshaw. Most outgrow the adversarial stage in adolescence and learn to appreciate their parents in young adulthood. However, for some, middle age is often the time that these issues once again come to the fore. Many struggle to let go of old parent–child battles, resentments, and hurts and go on with their lives. Midlife can offer another chance to finally get these issues resolved. Feeling deprived and needy, patients often vent angry feelings toward parents whom they feel were remiss in fulfilling their needs or did not love them enough.

Some try to handle their anger and resentment toward their parents by moving away. They may reduce their interactions this way, but geography does not solve the problem. The unresolved issues, the pain, and the tension remain. Only time and sincere effort on both parts can help. Some wrongly expect spouses or other people to fulfill the needs left unfulfilled from childhood. Such demands can put a strain on a marriage. The "child within" may have to learn that some deprivation cannot be fulfilled later in life. It may just have to be accepted. The area of deprivation will gradually heal over. It will always be a little thin—a little vulnerable.

For years, the feelings of deprivation will fester and periodically come to the surface. Being under stress for various reasons during midlife can make you feel needy. Once again, you will rework old frustrations. These fights with parents do nothing but prevent the anxious and insecure from facing the unknown and moving on. These interactions can serve a psychological purpose. As long as you battle away and hold on to this old anger, you do not have to grow up, take responsibility for yourself, or get on with your life. The following vignette will illustrate this point. Barbara's battle with her mother comes to the surface once again after she returns home to help her widowed mother cope with life after hip replacement surgery. As you will see, fortunately Barbara was able to put old tensions to rest and achieve a new emotional balance with her mother.

Vignette: Barbara and Her Mother

Barbara was 58 years old and she had been divorced for many years. Since the divorce, it was almost as if she had been hibernating. Her life had developed into a routine of working each day, seeing a few family members, and enjoying the peace and quiet of her small apartment. This routine changed abruptly three years ago when her father died. He had been an alcoholic and had separated from her mother many years before when Barbara was 16. Although the other family members hated him for his years of abusive behavior, Barbara loved him dearly. Prior to his death, she had taken care of him during nine months of a painful ordeal involving bone cancer. She felt that her mother resented her for doing so. Eighteen months later, her mother, who was gradually losing her sight, fell and broke a hip. Barbara moved in with her until she could once again take care of herself. "If I don't take care of Mom, I'll be a failure."

It was difficult for Barbara to return to her parents' house. She felt cramped in her old childhood room. The older woman balked if she tried to make changes in the house. Barbara resented the fact that her two younger siblings did not help out very much. She resented the negative things her mother said about her father. She still blamed her mother for the parental separation. The tension between them increased. In therapy, Barbara dealt with her image of what she had wanted her parents to be. Now that she had a second opportunity to get closer to her mother, she felt quite ambivalent. At first, she said that she resisted the intimacy because she would be left alone when her mother died. She dealt with her fears of being rejected. She complained that her mother sabotaged everything she did, and didn't appreciate her. Her

anger increased and the disagreements with her mother escalated. It
gradually became clear what was happening.

In a way, since moving home, Barbara was acting in two plays
at once. In one, she was a 58-year-old woman taking care of her 82-
year-old invalid mother. In the other, she was 16 again and filled with
all her old resentments. She had gone back to the point where she had
left off with her mother 42 years ago. Her mother, on the other hand,
was only dealing in the here and now. One night during therapy,
Barbara said, "Physically, I feel like a woman, but emotionally I'm a
girl." I asked her what age she felt like and what she wanted from her
mother. Instantly, she said 16, acceptance, and love. Barbara gradually
started to understand her recent emotionality. "Maybe this was God's
way of putting us together and allowing me to get closer to Mom." I
encouraged her to talk to her mother.

This was not an easy task. Barbara was filled with anger and
guilt. One night she took the risk. The words tumbled out as she
expressed her resentment that no matter what she did, her mother didn't
seem to feel she had done it right. She said that she was angry that
her brother and sisters didn't play their part in taking care of Mom.
Best of all, she told her mother how angry she had been at age 16,
when her mother had not allowed her to leave school and go to live
with her father when he had left. She felt that this meant her mother
resented her loving her father. Her mother explained the truth: she had
wanted Barbara to finish high school and live at home out of love and
concern, not out of anger or disapproval. "There's a little girl in me
who wants approval and someone to take care of me." Something started
to settle in Barbara. She felt as if she had achieved resolution and was
more at peace. For the first time, she began to see that her mother loved
her. She gradually started going out more and expanded her own life.

Acceptance and Appreciation

So often, patients see their parents only through their own
needs. How different they look when you take them off the
pedestal and see them as human beings with a life history and

needs of their own. Your parents may also have suffered emotional wounds and been deprived. They also had parents who raised them. How much easier it is to understand your parents' imperfections and appreciate their humanness when you see them from this more realistic vantage point. Many times, it is not until you have children of your own and have experienced some of life's trials and tribulations that you can start to understand and appreciate your parents. Perhaps at this juncture, you may realize for the first time that they were coming from a good place and really did do the best they could. If you try to understand their personalities and background, you may realize that contrary to prior belief, although not perfect, they did love, accept, and appreciate you.

I have seen many patients who carry a lopsided picture of their parents, which can affect their relationship and also how they feel about themselves. This is particularly an issue if the parent was highly critical or tended to deal with feelings in a loud, aggressive, or argumentative manner. The small child hears only the noisy giant adult and is not able to read between the lines and understand that the parents are perhaps only venting frustration. The child may grow up relating to only one aspect of the parents' personalities.

In doing therapy, I have heard many stories, for instance, of a child hiding under the table as an alcoholic father verbally abused a spouse or an older sibling. The child becomes frightened and anxious and may assume that she did something wrong. This behavior can also threaten the security of the child, who may be afraid his parents will leave or throw him out in the cold. Youngsters feel helpless and anxious because they have few resources outside the home. Many adults who have been brought up in this type of emotional atmosphere remain stymied as adults. It may take them some time, often through therapy, to realize that, as grownups, they have many resources and options.

Children may also react to the yelling by assuming that their parents do not love them. These false assumptions color their world and can cause internal conflicts which can sometimes come out in repetitive dreams or nightmares. Under such home conditions, children learn to protect themselves psychologically and may have difficulty dealing with their own feelings later on in life. Childhood behaviors may continue into adulthood, when they are no longer necessary, functional, or appropriate. This predicament is particularly relevant to the adult children of alcoholics, but is also seen in others.

Seeing your parents in a new light can do much to allow you to understand and accept yourself. Some say

> that men can soften the midlife blows by making a point to get to know their fathers, to understand the wounds that their fathers suffered—wounds that shaped the father–son relationships. Once a man understands his father, he is on the road toward understanding himself—because we truly are products of our upbringing. When we accept that the father did the best he could, considering his limitations, we can better accept ourselves and our limitations. That can free us to turn loose some of our defenses and to love more deeply.(5)

In my experience in doing therapy, these words certainly hold true for women also. In fact, understanding both of your parents as people can help you forgive, forget, mature, and grow.

Another childhood issue that may still fester in midlife has to do with sibling rivalry and notions of favoritism in reference to parental treatment. It is a myth that parents love all their children exactly the same. Although they may love all their children, differences in personalities, on both sides, do occur. Just as in other aspects of life, some personalities are more compatible. I have also seen cases in therapy where the child who is perceived as the strong one in the family (and who often then becomes the caretaker) feels unloved and neglected. The parent may indeed love the seemingly strong child, and often even think more of him or her. However, often the parent has paid or is still paying more attention toward another brother or sister whom they felt was either emotionally or physically weaker and needed their protection. The "stronger" child, now an adult, may have to learn to ask for what he or she wants. Understanding these dynamics can help put parent–child relationships in better perspective.

The final phase of midlife development is giving up the image of parents as being omnipotent and the childish expectation that they be perfect. If this process is successful, you will come to forgive your parents for their shortcomings, limitations, and mistakes and start to see them as they are or were: human, loving people who meant well and did the best they could. Hopefully, someday, your own children will return the favor by also understanding and forgiving you.(2)

The following vignette will illustrate some of these points. As Margie finally sees her father more clearly and accepts him warts and all, she is able to really understand and appreciate him. It also shows how Margie was able to feel more secure and believe more in her own self-worth once she started to see her father as human with both good and bad characteristics.

Vignette: Margie and Her Father

Margie was a whiz at work. She was efficient, knowledgeable, and hard working. Inside, though, she felt inadequate, insecure, and intellectually inferior. She complained that she had difficulty with her feelings and had a particularly hard time relating to men. She was concerned because she had just started a new relationship and wanted it to go well. She described her father as a strict, gruff man who always had to be right. "He yelled at me a lot. My feelings weren't acceptable. If I had feelings, I cried. I still do. I felt that if I didn't do everything he wanted, he wouldn't love me. The boys were encouraged to do well in school and could go out for team sports. I had to come right home from school and help Mom."

It had always been the same with men. "If there was a conflict with my brother, I gave in." Margie explained that she had walked on egg shells for 15 years in her own marriage. She finally left when her husband refused to let her return to work full time. When her father died, she was left feeling ambivalent and confused. "There was no closure. I felt left out. His death was somewhat of a release. He was so authoritarian. I had mixed feelings. I was never good enough."

Margie felt stressed both at work and in her new relationship. She seemed to be crying more. In therapy various themes repeated themselves. She spoke of people yelling at her, her upset with herself for becoming tearful, her need to please authority figures, and being intimidated by authority figures. She felt that her boyfriend did not value her opinions. Although she was 45 years old, she appeared much younger. One day in therapy, I could see that she very much wanted to say something and challenge my hypothesis. She didn't cry. Yet, she let me continue talking. When I asked her why, she stated that she had been taught that you don't interrupt grownups. We both laughed. She had no trouble interrupting me after that.

Another breakthrough came after I got her to talk about her father's good points. Prior to this session, I had only heard about the negative side of her father. Unexpectedly, she went on and on. She told me that he was helpful and that he could be counted on. He was mechanically inclined and liked to take trips. "He loved my mother very much and was affectionate to her." He was responsible, conscientious, and a good provider. He supported his church and taught at Sunday school. "He couldn't sleep until we got home." After this torrent of words, she sat quietly for a few moments, then said, "He had good and bad points, just like me!" For the first time, Margie thought of her father as being human. She had always seen him as all-powerful, strong, and not in the least vulnerable. She began to understand that her father's demeanor of being gruff and not complimentary toward her was just a facade. When she looked a little closer, it was obvious, 10 years after his death, that he had loved her. After this session, things began to go a little better for Margie.

Achieving a New Relationship

For some, midlife can bring a positive warm patina to parent–child relationships. The above discussion and vignettes are possible examples of what can happen. We tend to lean on the side of optimism and hope in therapy. Not everyone has a good relationship with their parents. Some parents may even be "toxic parents" who purposely try to knock down their children. You are not responsible for what happened in childhood. Even as an adult, you are only responsible for 50 percent of the relationship equation. You cannot retrain others. Someone else already brought your parents up. What really is possible in midlife probably falls on a continuum: some relationships improve and do well; others continue to be a mixture of love and hate, still others never improve or achieve a new balance; and many live with regrets and pain.

In any case, "as children begin to recognize their parents' strengths and weaknesses as individuals who have had numerous experiences, they begin to view them in a different way. That is, they begin to accept their parents rights, needs, and/or limitations."(6) This is bound to be beneficial. As noted above, acceptance can change the balance of your relationship with your mother and father in a positive direction. You will enjoy their company more and value your time together. Even if you do not choose to be closer, resolution of old problems can allow you to feel better about yourself and reduce guilt feelings. This new mutual respect can also allow you to move on with your life.

Sometimes change comes too late. For instance, a change or shift in feelings toward a parent coming after their death or after they have begun to deteriorate mentally can be a bittersweet accomplishment. Don't wait too long to work on your relationship or show your feelings. Too many adults still live by the adage that the parent is the older one and should make the first move. They may not be able to change. They may just not know how. If you want to share your positive feelings or make other changes, take a risk. Children are not the only ones who need love and attention. Older people also need and respond to affection, compliments, and love. Making peace with your parents will benefit you both.

Mom and Dad Are Getting Old: How About Me?

Realizing that your parents are aging has to affect you. Just as other milestones and turning points do, this awareness forces you to see that time has passed and that you also are older. For some, this is a gradual process. For others, this transition can come with a thud. In any case, change in your parents' health and vitality is another landmark that will cause you to evaluate your own life in middle age and add to the "midlife crisis." It will also make you think of future obligations and responsibilities. In a practical sense, it can force you to think about your parents' future needs, open discussions with them, and make tentative plans. It also underlines that fact that life has limits.

A theme that recurs in therapy is the patient who is overly worried about his or her parents' dying. Often this can be interpreted symbolically rather than literally. These patients are often really worried about themselves and their ability to be independent. They are usually quite anxious about their ability to cope with the future, its responsibilities, and its unknown quality. They are really saying, "I am not ready to grow up and replace my parents in the adult world." At times, this concern, if it becomes obsessive, can also mask other worries or feelings. This possibility should be explored.

Facing Your Own Mortality

Coming to terms with one's own mortality has been called the central task of midlife. We all carry the illusion of immortality and usually try consciously not to think about death. In middle age this gets harder to do. The inevitability of death becomes a more consciously perceived threat. You realize that you are closer to the end of life than you are to the beginning. Parents and relatives retire, become ill, and die. Colleagues and friends your own age suddenly collapse and are gone. You start to notice the physical signs of aging in yourself. In midlife, "the blinders of youth drop away, and you realize that life has not just a beginning, but also an end."(7) I recently had lunch with a friend who related that a neighbor's parent had just died. "It got me thinking," he said. "We're the next generation. The next to go."

Elliott Jacques, who is credited with having coined the term "midlife crisis" explored the psychology of middle age in his article, "Death and the Midlife Crisis."(8) He felt that in midlife the nature of creativity changes to tragic, reflective, more conservative and philosophical themes brought on by the inevitability of death. "In the mature adult," he says, "idealism is given up and supplemented by a more contemplative pessimism." Thus, midlife death anxiety can inhibit creativity. This may only be one possibility. It may also inspire a phoenixlike creativity that is life affirming.(9)

Many patients are concerned about death. They may worry about it, avoid talking about it, or use euphemisms or synonyms to describe it. However, since we really do not know what death is, perhaps they are really worried about the unknown. The fear of death is really the fear of the unknown—of Hamlet's "undiscovered country." Death is a universal experience which must be confronted and accepted as inevitable. Those who have strong religious convictions and conceive of life after death can find comfort in these beliefs. We know from observation of those dying from a terminal illness that dying is a process. The coping responses during this period "are shaped by previous experiences with death, as well as by cultural attitudes and beliefs. In essence, one tends to die as one has lived."(10)

The Loss of a Parent

Dealing with the death of a parent is not just saying goodbye. It is a process of mourning and hopefully of continued development and growth. For some, it is a time to deal with old issues and feelings of resentment. It may be a time of dealing with guilt. For others, it can be time of knowing that they did everything they could; a time to cherish the good memories which no one can ever take away. If you have been successful in putting the negative in perspective, your good memories and the positive impact of your parents' personality will stay with you and comfort you forever. On another positive note, the death of a parent is a process that can end in a feeling of increased autonomy as you truly take over the parent's role and replace him or her. After the initial period of mourning, you can gradually go on to achieve a sense of new fulfillment as you become one of the elders and provide wisdom and guidance to others.

After a loss, mourning and grief is a normal process. It is not a sign of weakness or self-indulgence. The healing process after a major loss, such as the death of a parent, will take some time and varies from person to person. It is normal to think about the lost person and become tearful and briefly distraught at times, particularly on their birthday, or on the anniversary of their death. For some children, the death of a parent will be a tremendous loss, leaving them feeling helpless and alone. Those who usually have the most difficulty are those who have mixed or ambivalent feelings about the parent due to anger or disappointment. However, as a general rule of thumb, if you are still exhibiting signs of major distress and not functioning well after three months, it may be helpful to talk to your physician. You may be suffering from a clinical depression rather than just responding normally to this life event. (See Chapter 9 for symptoms of a clinical depression.)

The classic work of Kübler-Ross(11) provides a framework for understanding the dynamics of the grieving process. She elaborates five stages that summarize the behaviors and feelings associated with the death of a parent or significant other: denial, anger, bargaining, depression, and acceptance. Kübler-Ross stresses that acceptance is coming to terms with the situation rather than resignation or hopelessness. At this point the grieved will return to their prior level of functioning and resume their normal personal, social, and work interactions. These same stages will be experienced by those who are facing a physical deformity or their own death.

Guidelines for Success

- *Believe in yourself.* Look at what you have accomplished. Give yourself some credit. Don't be afraid to take independent action or try new behavior.
- *Let go of old anger and resentment.* These feelings are self-defeating and self-destructive. They can only use up energy and bog you down. Reduce your inappropriate guilt. You are not responsible for what happened when you were a child.
- *You are not helpless.* You may just feel that way now because you felt that way when you were a child. Realize that as an adult, you have many resources and options that were not available to you earlier in life.
- *Continue to work on your relationship with your parents.* Each interaction can be a new beginning. Making peace with your parents will benefit you both.
- *Refuse to jump into the ring and fight.* You can change the subject or limit the interaction.
- *Learn as much as you can about your parents' background and history.* Particularly helpful will be information about traumatic events and the people who helped mold them. Understanding their wounds will help you forgive and forget.
- *Talk to someone if you need help in understanding your parents' personalities.* You may not be seeing the whole picture. You may need to purge the anger, the hurt, and resentment before you can understand and forgive.
- *Accept yourself and your parents as imperfect human beings.* You both have good and bad points. Be more compassionate. It's hard to make peace with yourself if you are not able to make peace with your parents.

- *Face the unknown.* It may be positive. Change can be good.
- *Life is short.* Be kind to one another.

In becoming a parent to your parents, you must learn to deal with new situations and new feelings. This process can be rewarding as you renew mutual love and appreciation. Sometimes, in caring for aging parents, there is also ambivalence, guilt, and resentment, as well as satisfaction. The next two chapters will present an overview of the parent–child relationship at the other end of the rainbow and look at some of the changes both in their lives and in yours that can occur during their golden years as you become a middle-aged caregiver.

Part IV

THE TRADITIONAL GENERATION

Chapter 11

The Golden Years

Late adulthood begins at approximately 60 to 65 years of age. During this period, senior citizens, confronted with the emotional and physical demands and changes of old age, face new challenges in coping with life. There is no one stereotype to describe this time of life. Chronology aside, we all move through life on different biological, social, and psychological tracks. What happens during the "golden years" will depend on the tone and achievements of prior developmental phases. There is no time limit to psychological growth and development. "The major developmental task of old age is to find, clarify, and deepen what one has attained from a lifetime of learning and adapting."(1) Other developmental tasks of senior adulthood include adjusting to physical aging, decreasing physical strength, and declining health; adjusting to retirement and living on a fixed, reduced, income; coping with the death of a spouse and/or the death of loved ones; establishing new living arrangements and establishing relationships with people of the same age.(2)

According to Erikson(3), the challenge of old age or the final stage of man is "integrity versus despair." A sense of emotional integrity is derived from an individual's overall satisfaction with life. If the individual has no regrets over the past and views his or her life as meaningful, he or she potentially can accept the future with equanimity. A life history characterized by personal trust, a sense of autonomy, initiative, a solid identity, intimacy, and generativity will lead naturally in the later years to a sense of integrity and an acceptance of death. The individual who lacks this integration and sees life as a series of missed opportunities is likely to be discontented and despair over the realization that it is too late to start over. The sense that time is running out combined with the feeling that one has not lived fully causes fear of facing death.(2,4)

Having burst the illusion of invincibility and immortality, "the adult beyond midlife demonstrates a progressive interiority, an inner acceptance of his or her own values, less social posturing, fewer defensive strategies, [decreased internal tension, and a feeling of steadiness], and in general, more of an attitude of 'Here I am world, take it or leave it. No apologies!' "(5)

As noted, people differ in their ability to adapt to the challenges of aging. The first test of their resiliency may be retirement. Let's look at this plateau through the eyes of George, who in his sixties learns that life doesn't always turn out the way we planned.

Vignette: George

George had looked forward to retirement for many years. The long-awaited day finally came six months ago, complete with farewell speeches and a gold watch. For a while, he was happy with his new-found freedom. He could sleep late and didn't have to deal with schedules, company meetings, and the constant tension of the large manufacturing plant that had been his life for 33 years. Lately, though, everything had changed. His wife, Ethel, always neat and punctual, seemed to resent his presence in "her house" and his small demands on her time. Trivial arguments seemed to be the norm. The day seemed long as he moped and puttered in his small garden. Somehow, he missed the hustle and bustle of his old job. No one came to him for decisions any longer. He had always been a good provider, but now he worried silently about his being able to exist on a fixed income. His body seemed to hurt in new places. He felt isolated, alone, and rudderless. The neat rows of vegetables were growing beautifully. His neighbors envied his leisure.

His daughter, Mary, called faithfully each Sunday from California. Why wasn't it enough? Why wasn't George happy?

Growing older and retiring isn't always easy. Many like George and Ethel will experience pain and frustration born of their own difficulties in dealing with change and the accentuation of their own personality traits. For some, work or family is the only investment they have made in life. When physical illness and lowered economic status are added, they feel helpless and useless. For those who have planned ahead by developing other interests and hobbies, the later years can be a time of joy and contentment. People who have self-assertive problem-solving approaches to life do best. For them, retirement will be a time to expand life in new directions and develop new outlooks and interests.(6)

The key to a successful retirement is to stay involved. It is important to have something to get up for in the morning and something to look forward to. Keep busy. Continue to learn and grow. Continue to share your knowledge and teach the younger generation. Look to the future with optimism. Retain a passion for work or other projects. Continue to invest yourself in others. This will help you to continue to feel needed and alive and fill your life with meaning.(7) Many have never been able to achieve these goals and may continue to have difficulty in retirement.

Coping with a Retired Parent

It is difficult to change or undo a lifetime of habits or personality traits. However, if your parent is retired and unhappy, you will be concerned. Be supportive. Let the retiree know that you care and need him or her. Encourage him or her to try new things. More specifically, if Mom or Dad seem to be foundering with their new freedom and extra time after retirement, here are a few things you can do to help. However, remember that in the end, it is their responsibility to change and solve their dilemma.

Explore community resources. So many events and activities are available in the average community. There are sights to see, entertainment possibilities, sporting events, and interesting shops and restaurants to explore. Museums and movies often give senior discounts. There are clubs for almost everything from outdoor activities to playing bridge. Churches and synagogues have senior citizen groups that are always pleased to have new members. Community mental health centers often have senior programs that offer lunch and four hours of activities. If your parents are normally not too assertive or adventuresome, it may be difficult to get them to go, but don't stop trying. I once had a patient I encouraged to join a senior center group for almost a year. She finally went for one visit. She now goes five days a week.

Encourage them to try new things. Hobby possibilities abound. Like George, your parents may have an interest in gardening. I once had an elderly patient in her nineties who, walking with a cane, still tramped through her tomato garden each morning, enjoyed pulling out a few weeds, and took great pride in her yearly crop. If Mom or Dad don't seem to have any ideas, encourage new activity by helping them reach back and remember. Perhaps they can renew an old interest. Ask them about things they either did when they were younger or wanted to do and didn't have the time. What were their hopes and dreams when they were adolescents? These questions may get them thinking, light a spark, and open up new avenues.

As we shall see, the senior years can be a time of great creativity. Your parents may want to take art lessons or try some craft. If they collected stamps at age 10, they may enjoy collecting commemoratives today. If they always wanted to play the piano, they may be able to take a course at the local high school educational night. I knew a man in his eighties who decided to learn Italian so that he could visit Italy, a lifelong dream. Nostalgia itself can become a hobby, as the senior collects items or listens to old radio shows on cassette. The local library may be a source of information.

Work. For some the answer may be a parttime job. This can be invigorating for many seniors but is particularly helpful for those whose lives revolved around the marketplace. Possible positions may include substitute teaching, baby sitting, or clerking at a local store. A patient of mine was able to get parttime employment as a substitute lunch-room aid for a school district. Seniors bring with them a surplus of knowledge and good judgment that is often appreciated by an employer. Working even parttime will give them something to wake up for and look forward to. They will also value the small income such jobs can generate and still not interfere with their social security benefits.

Professional people, such as lawyers, physicians, and accountants, can often continue to work parttime, teach, or do consulting work. Artists, painters, sculptors, musicians, and writers can continue to enjoy their craft as long as they are physically and mentally able. Many can recycle their skills in new arenas. An accountant or businessman may enjoy being a treasurer or a consultant for a small business or organization.

Volunteerism. Helping others can give much satisfaction and help increase self-esteem. Hospitals, schools, and nursing homes often encourage and delight in having able-bodied older adults lend a helping hand. Many such programs allow you to work a few hours each week and often have an awards luncheon each year. Fraternal, religious, and philanthropic organizations or agencies also welcome participation by people of all ages.

Family involvement. Some older adults are perfectly content just being at home. However, they will appreciate being needed. They want to continue to invest themselves in and care for others. They may enjoy offering a helping hand with their grandchildren. This may include babysitting to give you a break or filling in until you return from work. Just be sure that they are really willing and not just feeling pressured or obligated. Remember to do something nice for them also. As you and your children get older, grandparents continue to get much pride in sharing family occasions and celebrations. Remember to include them whenever possible. As we shall see, being a grandparent can be a delight.

Travel. There is a whole world out there to explore. Various possibilities exist for every budget. Elderhostel, the American Association of Retired Persons, and others offer many group opportunities. Ask your travel agent about senior discounts and ways to get around the single supplement. Just planning a trip can give many pleasurable hours of reviewing travel possibilities and looking at travel brochures. I knew a 90-year-old man who was going to night school to learn Italian so he could visit the land of his birth.

Encourage involvement with others. Suggest ways that your parents can decrease isolation and increase their support system. Both will help reduce feelings of depression and help renew feelings of self-esteem. All of the suggestions above will encourage them to get involved and help in this direction. Don't forget resources in your own backyard. A patient of mine came alive when her daughter introduced her to her friend's widowed mother. Both women enjoyed the companionship and looked forward to their visits together. If they are interested, an introduction to a senior of the opposite sex is appreciated.

Even though you may want to help, there is a limit to what you can do to help your retired parents adjust. Sometimes even though they complain, they may really be content in their discontent and are just venting frustration. If such is the case, just listen and don't try to change the situation. This is particularly true if the complaints involve their marital situation. Couples tend to reach a certain equilibrium. It is not always the noisy one who is the problem; each is responsible for 50 percent of the marital interaction. For instance, if one is more active or assertive than the other, you may feel sorry for the parent who is left behind or seems upset by being dragged along. This may really represent ingrained patterns. The quiet one may have to be more assertive about his or her needs and desires. Certainly encourage each partner individually, but do not get in the middle of the relationship. If one partner seems lonely, you may wish to include him or her a little more in your own life.

You can encourage, gently prod, and suggest a few alternatives. However, do not attempt to solve it for them. It is their life. Try to be more objective and don't impose your own agenda. Some may be fiercely independent and have a need to do it themselves. Some are resistant because they are frightened. They will have to make changes at their own pace as they gain confidence. You may also have to accept the fact that even though your suggestions seem excellent, your advice won't always be taken. At times, you may have to realize that even though you are concerned and care, all they really may need is your interest and love.

Grandparenthood

There is one thing that you can do to add dimension and happiness to your parents' later years. Have children. Regardless of their level of content or discontent in the other areas of their life, grandparenting is a guaranteed pleasure. Ask an older person about their grandchildren and they tend to beam with pride. It works both ways. Grandparents are special people to their grandchildren. In doing therapy, I will often ask about various significant people in the patient's upbringing. Sometimes, parents and others will bring only a flicker of emotion. Ask about grandparents, however, and you often see a light bulb of positive feelings come on. As the child is growing up, grandparents often give unconditional love as well as providing a sense of family continuity and a perspective on an earlier era.

Grandparenthood can be a new lease on life. Except for the few who see it as a threat of approaching death, it allows a sense of psychological immortality and biological continuation with the future. It allows the experience of parenthood from a special perspective, one step removed, without parental responsibilities or stresses. More relaxed and confident, and in a new stage of life themselves, senior citizens may be able to enjoy and interact more with their grandchildren than they did their own children. It can provide a sense of emotional self-fulfillment. It offers a new role as teacher and resource person.(8)

Grandparents are not always older and retired like George and Ethel. Grandparenthood is likely to occur during midlife, when work and other involvement is still at its peak. Many thirtysomething children today, looking for help with their children, often ask, "What ever happened to all the old-fashioned grandmothers?" Young widowed grandmothers, busy with their own lives, may avoid or resent requests to care for their grandchildren. They often do not see babysitting as pleasurable or part of their role. They are sometimes pleased to return to the quiet of their own home and get back to their own routine. Grandparents may differ in both age and style. Styles may range from the formal grandparent, the grandparent as reservoir of family wisdom, the distant grandparent, to the fun-seeking grandparent. Some grandparents will assume child-care responsibilities for a parent who works and actually become a surrogate parent.(9)

Creativity in Late Life

> It is too late!
> Ah, nothing is too late
> till the tired heart shall
> cease to palpitate.
> For age is opportunity
> no less
> Than youth itself,
> though in another dress
> and as the evening
> twilight fades away

The sky is filled with stars,
invisible by day.

HENRY WADSWORTH LONGFELLOW
Morituri Salutamus (1875)

Wonderful things can continue to happen in late life. Older adults bring a lifetime of wisdom and experience to all they touch. Immersion in creative activity can bring additional meaning to their lives. Although creativity usually indicates the arts or writing, in discussing the emergence of creativity in late life, I will use the term "creativity" in the broadest sense to include any productive and satisfying activity or behavior, including new career/work involvement, volunteer activity, or even the expansion of meaningful relationships.

Creativity in the elderly can be developed in various ways. It can represent an important part of the person's life that began in childhood or adolescence and was nurtured consistently throughout life. Some individuals—for example, Rembrandt, Picasso, Michelangelo, Beethoven, and Bach—surpassed themselves as they grew older, reinforcing the phrase "not older, but better." Creative geniuses such as Aristotle and Freud continued to progress almost in parallel with their life course. Many contemporary men and women continued brilliant careers in the arts far into their senior years. Examples include Marc Chagall, Martha Graham, Eugene Ormandy, and Ruth Gordon.(10) Thomas Edison continued his experiments into late life, and Harvey Firestone and Henry Ford continued to do business in the usual way.

Creativity in the later years can also be a response to loss and loneliness. The deficit situation may be social isolation due to the loss of well-established social networks after moving to a new environment or due to chronic illness. It can also result from emotional isolation due to the loss of meaningful intimate relationships. As the social network decreases in size, the formation of new emotional bonds becomes more difficult. Women, particularly, may at this time experience a reawakening of previous artistic endeavors, such as creative writing and painting, left behind earlier in life because of caregiving and parenting obligations. Volunteer work can add something new to life and be a creative response to both emotional and social isolation.

Finally, creativity can be an entirely new endeavor begun in older age. Women, in particular, turn to creative writing in their later years to satisfy their generative needs. It has been suggested that perhaps writing does not require practice over the years, as do other talents such as music and art. Often, writing, in this age group, appears to be an attempt to master Erikson's last stage of life-span development, *integrity*. Autobiographical works at this age may be a way to make things right or leave something for posterity. Some continue to write after this original impulse is satisfied.(11) Even persons who do not have a gift for work or artistic talents can respond to the needs of their later years with "creative living," continuing to invest themselves in other people and meaningful activities. This can be good advice but difficult to follow, especially after the death of a spouse.

To Live Again: Life after the Death of a Spouse

The death of a spouse is the one life event that ranks highest on the social readjustment rating scale. One can anticipate and plan for many other life changes, but what do you do when your spouse suddenly is gone and you are left alone with your feelings and multiple responsibilities? Even if you can deal with all of this, where do you go from there? At best, life after death of a spouse is a difficult and stressful time. The sudden change in the widowed person's lifestyle creates strong spiritual and emotional needs during a time when they may have to deal with complex legal and financial transactions and start to plan a new future without their spouse.

People differ in their response to this situation. The death of a spouse during middle age appears to be more stressful than a similar loss later in life. Studies have shown that older widows adjust more easily than younger ones.(12) The impact of the spouse's death also depends on the importance of the marriage role for the survivor and the degree of closeness of the partners. The situation may not be as devastating for those whose identity was based more on career involvement or parenthood or for those who tolerated an unhappy marriage.(9)

In 1984, while doing my American Cablevision television show, "Mental Notes with Dr. Michael Zal," I had occasion to meet and interview members of a local group called To Live Again (TLA)(13). TLA had been formed in 1973 by a group of five recently widowed persons who felt that it would be helpful to have an empathetic friend or guide to meet the needs for support and guidance of the recently widowed on a nonprofessional level. Their philosophy and goals are based on the hypothesis that the widowed will never become their own selves again, but can emerge as different, but complete, persons capable of loving, giving, and living again. They further felt that the widowed who have learned to live again must share their strength, faith, and hope with those still struggling with grief.

TLA underscores the fact that grief is an inevitable and fitting reaction and tribute to the loss of something very precious. Grief is not a sign of weakness. "Let grief have its way for a while," they say, "and gradually and gently it will release you from its grip." They further maintain that most people go through a pattern of grief, not necessarily through all stages, nor in the same order. As noted in Chapter 10, according to Kübler-Ross, people go through various characteristic stages following the death of a loved one. The men and women of TLA, who have been there, expand on this concept specifically in reference to the loss of a spouse and say that the grief cycle consists of the following stages:

1. State of shock
2. Express emotions (and correct false beliefs)
3. Depression and loneliness
4. Physical symptoms and distress
5. Panic and disbelief

6. Sense of guilt
7. Hostility, resentment, and anger
8. Inability to return to usual activities
9. Hope comes through
10. Affirm reality about yourself

In my experience with people in therapy, it usually takes a full year for a widow or widower to form a new life, feel whole again, and truly start to live again. Along the way there will be bumps, hard times, anniversary reactions, and private moments of sadness, fear, and loneliness. Most at risk is the widow whose sorrow is mixed with feelings of fear and helplessness. During her marriage, she never had anything to do with the financial or business aspects of her life. Her spouse, feeling he was doing his duty, kept all such information to himself and took care of everything. He did not do his spouse a favor by this overprotective attitude. Such widows will have to gain confidence in making decisions and learning to take care of their own needs. I have seen such women struggle desperately to establish their own identities and feelings of competence. For these women, "even the death of a deeply loved partner can have its positive aspects. Many such individuals come to realize for the first time that they do possess the personal strength and resources to cope with any and all of life's vicissitudes."(9)

Another group who may have difficulty and suffer a prolonged grief reaction are those who had ambivalent feelings about their spouses. With such persons, tearfulness and agitation may last for months after the event. Although it may be hard to express, some will be angry that their spouses died and left them with all the responsibility. Others will harbor much self-pity or unexpressed, pent-up anger and resentment over past unfulfilled needs. Some will carry an undue burden of guilt and feel that they should have done more. At another extreme is the 80-year-old woman who came to me due to a depression following the death of her third husband. After several weeks of therapy, when she was starting to feel a little better, she said, "I've been here before. I know what I have to do [to go on with her life], but I just don't feel like doing it again."

Various problems may arise. The new widow or widower will have to deal with the loss of friends as people no longer call and married friends see them as a threat to their own spouse now that they are single. They will have to make new friends, change their lifestyle, sell a family home and possessions, or perhaps go back to work. Each step can mean new anxiety and pain. Although there are many roadblocks to achieving emotional peace, contentment, understanding, and acceptance, most will take a problem-solving approach, meet the challenge, and arrive at that day. They will make new discoveries along the way about themselves, others, and the world. They will become stronger and gain confidence in the process. The widow or widower will realize that they will be left with their good memories, which will always be theirs and can never be taken away. Time does heal. The grief will end and they will start to live again.

Sex after Sixty

A significant link in the chain of mythology surrounding the senior citizen is the fallacy that older men and women are nonsexual. "Desexualizing people as soon as they qualify for Social Security is a popular tendency. However, sexual activity and interest, as well as the need for affection and companionship, certainly continue long after age 65."(6) Sexual love can contribute to the well-being of older couples. "If one is healthy and has an interested and interesting partner, sexual desire, ability, and satisfaction can continue throughout life."(1)

Age does bring some modification in sexual responsiveness. The aging man achieves erection more slowly. He may require his partner to provide more stimulation but may be too proud or embarrassed to ask. His wife may also have to be more active in assisting him in entering the vagina if he is not achieving a complete erection. Men who are sexually inactive can become impotent. Older women may have a reduction in the number of orgasmic contractions. They may find sexual intercourse uncomfortable and even painful due to shortening, a decrease in expansibility, and thinning of the walls of the vagina. There will be a loss of natural lubrication due to depleted estrogen stores. The use of a sterile lubricant, such as K-Y jelly, available over the counter at the drugstore, can be helpful. As they grow older, couples may experience a decline in their sexual interest, but the timing and rate of decline may be different for each partner. A man and wife who were sexually compatible earlier in life may encounter difficulty after 60.(6,14)

The elderly person may be having sexual problems for various other reasons. They may be losing interest due to boredom with the same partner, mental and physical fatigue, fear of performance failure, and overindulgence in alcohol and food. Many suffer from chronic illness such as diabetes, heart disease, emphysema, and arthritis, which may be affecting their sexuality. Medications, such as antihypertensives, tranquilizers and sedatives, antidepressants, antihistamines, and anticholinergics, can interfere with sexual physiology and produce dysfunction.(15) It is best to ask your family physician or pharmacist if you have questions about these possible interactions. Given the opportunity, most elderly people welcome the chance to talk to an understanding and accepting person about their sexuality.

"Often, the attitudes of others influence sexual matters in the elderly. Children, other family members, and helping professionals may sometimes have to be reassured that the continued sexual behavior of their charges is normal and healthy."(6) Most families maintain a wall of silence about sexual issues. It is okay if you talk to your parents about sex. Try to maintain a positive attitude. Watch your language. People of different generations have different sensitivities about sexual words. Don't assume that your parents know how you feel. Be direct and open. If you do not think what they are doing is right, tell them but tell them why. But do not assume you have the right to make decisions for them.(14)

This may be particularly an issue in a nursing-home setting, where residents may wish to walk together, hold hands, or even spend the night together. In this setting, rooms are segregated by sex and administrators often look aghast at any suggestion that their charges have sexual and/or affectional needs. In fact, no activity has greater potential for both physical and psychological reassurance than sexuality. Nothing has more of a capacity to reinforce the feeling of being a desired, meaningful, man or woman.(16) Male–female companionship can add to the quality of one's life throughout adulthood.

It is a new world out there. Attitudes are changing. Social barriers to sex after 60 are lifting. More information is available. Older people no longer have to suppress sexual interest as much due to disapproval or the possibility that it will be seen by others as being grotesque. Men and women are living together after 65 without marriage in order not to lose Social Security benefits. Some couples live apart but travel together on vacation, introducing themselves to friends and new acquaintances as "this is my live-in" or significant other. "The benefits of sharing an intimate relationship are often sufficient to override guilt feelings, family disapproval, or other negative reactions."(16) Being loved and cared for are important needs at any age.

We are learning that the elderly are human beings and that it is helpful to understand them in their totality. The common misconception of old age as being a time of second childhood when the individual becomes feeble in mind and body is not true. Most people age comfortably and in good health. Physical, psychosocial, and economic factors are all important to a full understanding of the dynamics and unique problems of the senior citizen. Each stage of life has its own set of problems and rewards. Persons who by personality have taken a problem-solving approach to life will do well. For them the later years will be a time of joy and contentment. They have planned ahead and developed interests and hobbies outside the realm of work or raising a family, If they are lucky, physical illness or lowered economic status will not take their toll.

For others, the picture may be different. For these persons, the later years may be a time of frustration. They may experience pain born of their own difficulties in dealing with change and the accentuation of their own personality traits. Some will be involved in a battle over change in residence, wills, and other financial matters, or business responsibilities. For many, physical illness or the death of a friend or family member will be a tremendous loss, leaving them feeling helpless and alone. Most, however, will fall between these two extremes. All in all, the [1990s] are a time of hope and promise for the senior citizen. Growing older in the [1990s] can be an enjoyable and special experience.(6)

When does the mature adult or senior citizen become old? It is hard to pinpoint. There is always a gradual transition from one stage to another. One really has to take into account prior life history, including personality traits, environmental stress, and general health, as well as chronological age. As a physician, I see many "old old" people, over age 85, who are still functioning well and enjoying life. However, repeated losses and physical change can take their toll. We all reach the end of the line. Some become frail and dependent. The next chapter will deal with some of the issues that the vulnerable older individual must cope with as well as some of the complex problems you may have to face as a caregiver to the elderly.

Chapter 12

The Last Mile

Vignette: Emma

Emma is old but not dead, although to some she is invisible. She sits passive but resolute in "her seat" in the lobby of the retirement home. She has been at her post daily for the past 15 months since her family decided that they could no longer care for her in their home. Her arthritic fingers pick aimlessly at the fabric of her soiled housedress on her broad lap. Her eyes, sad and bored, watch carefully the familiar dull events of the day. Her mind, remembering the past more clearly than the present, settles for a moment on happier days when she felt useful and needed. People come and go, unaware of her presence. Other residents seem lost in their own thoughts and memories. An occasional visitor moves quickly out of her limited range of vision. She brightens perceptibly as a familiar face passes, calls her name, and waves hello. Emma may be confused but she senses the interest and emotion in the voice and action. She smiles for the first time in many days.

We will all grow older. You would think that this fact alone would give each of us tremendous empathy and compassion for the elderly such as Emma. However, in a society that worships youthfulness, health, and vitality, the needs and concerns of senior citizens are often forgotten and ignored. Many would like the elderly to become invisible. Some professionals share this bias and are reluctant to treat the elderly patient because they wrongly feel that nothing can be done. Other cultures have different attitudes toward the elderly, which improve their quality of life in later years. The Chinese seem to revere their elders for their wisdom and experience. In India, also, people have a tremendous sense of duty and responsibility toward their relatives. Elderly people are honored as symbols of humanity and divinity and they are held in the highest esteem.(1)

Our attitudes will have to change. The population in the United States is growing older. People are living longer due to improved public health, new lifesaving medical technologies, and perhaps a decrease in smoking and drinking. The number of the elderly in the United States will double in the next 50 years. The United States Census Bureau estimates that more than 30 million people are age 65 or older, representing more than 12 percent of the country's population. This compares to 3 percent of the population in 1900. By the year 2000, 20 percent of Americans will be senior citizens age 65 or older. At present, 12.5 million are over 75, and nearly 3 million are over 85.(2) This last group, often frail and disabled, now constitutes what we call the "old old" generation. In the next decade, they are expected to grow 42 percent, up to at least 4.6 million people. By the year 2040, they could easily reach 45 million.(3) As the population matures, we will all need knowledge and understanding of the elderly. Only an informed lay and professional population can help formulate new solutions to the problems of aging.

Understanding the Elderly

"A stumbling block to our realistic understanding of the elderly is the misconception that senility is the only problem of the aged. When many think of the elderly, the confused, forgetful, childlike person comes to mind. In reality, however, most are competent, active, and alert. Most people age comfortably and in good health. The organic brain syndrome, or dementia, a complex of brain disorders caused by the impairment of brain tissue function, is found in only about 15 percent of people past age

55—a decided minority." According to the American Psychiatric Association Division of Public Affairs, nearly one-fourth of the elderly who are labeled senile actually suffer some form of mental illness that can be effectively treated. "The elderly are prone to a full range of emotional or functional problems, including neurotic symptoms, personality disorders, and even psychotic syndromes. Drug and alcohol abuse often are hidden disorders in this age group. Many people develop a habitation to sleeping pills, pain medication, tranquilizers, or other favorite medications.

"Who is not aware that bowel function and digestion are often a preoccupation of the elderly? As people become more narcissistic or self-centered with age, they turn their energy from the external world to themselves. However, despite this normal preoccupation, true hypochondriacal physical complaints are often common and can mask other symptoms, especially depression. This is a difficult differential. However, the complaints of the elderly should be taken seriously. An old wives' tale claims that older people need less sleep than do younger people. The opposite is true. Sleep disturbances at this age are pathognomonic of psychic disturbance."(1) The major psychiatric illnesses of old age are Alzheimer's disease and depression. Let's look more closely at these two disorders.

Dementia

Dementia means loss of mental powers due to impairment of brain tissue function. The term comes from the Latin meaning "away + the mind."(4) The organic brain disorders describe a group of illnesses, caused by structural damage or destruction in the brain. These changes cause a gradual but persistent deterioration of neurological and psychological functioning characterized by symptoms of impairment of orientation (to time, place, and person) and memory, particularly of immediate recall. Changes in intellectual functioning will also occur, including difficulty in performing simple calculations, recalling simple items of general information, comprehending, and retaining and reacting to questions and commands. These disorders are also prone to show lability and shallowness of affect, as well as impairment of judgment. The organic mental disorders can be grouped into three categories.

Reversible brain syndromes, also called acute brain syndromes, are transient, potentially reversible conditions that are "usually related to acute febrile, debilitating, or exhausting illness. The underlying factors may be malnutrition, infection, fractures, heart failure, drug interactions, malignancy, electrolyte imbalance, metabolic disorders, vomiting, renal disease, or even emotional overreaction. The first order of business in treating these patients is to correct the underlying and causative conditions which are amenable to treatment."(5) Twenty percent of dementias are reversible.(6)

Alzheimer's Disease, first described by German psychiatrist Alois Alzheimer in 1907, is a chronic, irreversible, progressive deterioration of brain cells which accounts for 40 to 60 percent of dementias. The cause is unknown and remains an unsolved medical puzzle. Research possibilities include increased aluminum in the brain, inappropriate levels of the brain enzyme choline acetyltransferase, or a slow-acting virus. There is no specific treatment at present although many of the associated symptoms can be eased with medication. Psychotherapy can be of some value with an organic patient, even if he or she does not seem to comprehend the intervention. The presence of the therapist often hits an emotional note and results in a more cooperative and responsive patient. Family members will also require counseling and emotional support. Primary degenerative dementia of the Alzheimer's type is inherited. The odds of developing Alzheimer's disease increase fourfold among family members of a person suffering from the disorder.

Multi-infarct dementia is the second most common cause of irreversible dementia. It is caused by small strokes that gradually produce a loss of brain tissue due to insufficient circulation to the affected areas of the brain. It is associated with high blood pressure and usually progresses in a step-like pattern of symptoms interspersed with long periods of stable functioning. The pattern of deficits is "patchy" depending on which regions of the brain have been destroyed. Focal neurologic signs may also be present, such as weakness in the limbs, reflex changes, changes in gait, and changes in speech.

> The clinical course in . . . these syndromes is usually variable and fluctuating. At times you may observe a quiet individual who seems to be cooperative and functioning; at other times, this same individual may be restless, helpless, bewildered, and confused with physical and verbal wandering. He or she may whine or cry. Such behavior often causes frustration and concern in those caring for the patient in nursing homes and hospitals. Often the emotional lability is interpreted as clinical depression. Family members are often concerned that their confused, tearful, senile relative is unhappy and suffering; however, the patient may actually experience little, if any, subjective suffering.(5)

Vignette: Sallie

Sallie lay huddled in her hospital bed, unable to sleep, weeping silently into her pillow. Her gray hair, wet from her tears, fell into her reddened eyes. She had suffered a stroke but was doing well medically. She recently learned to transfer herself from bed to wheelchair and felt proud of her newfound freedom. Her physical loss was great but other losses disturbed her more. An older sister, whom she had relied on as a mother, had died months before. Her husband had died the year before. During her hospitalization, her worldly possessions had been stolen. Although Sallie's remaining family members had been supportive at first, they now visited infrequently. She wanted to be independent but felt helpless and irritable. The doctors told her she had to start a new life. She also knew that she would have to spend many months in a rehabilitation center before she could once again return to her empty home. She wanted to try but it felt like forever just to get to tomorrow. Depressed and alone, she gradually drifted into a troubled sleep.(1)

Depression in the Elderly

Sallie illustrates the most common psychiatric reaction in the geriatric population. Clinical depression afflicts up to 5 percent of people aged 65 or older although some epidemiologic estimates range up to 50 percent. The highest suicide rate in the United States is among this age group.(7) Depression is a reaction to loss and change. Although not always as pervasive as Sallie's situation, the elderly do suffer losses in many areas.

Forgetfulness and impairment in cognitive ability produce psychologic losses. Physical and physiologic losses follow changes in health, strength, and appearance. Economic losses are caused by reduced income, property loss, and employment reduction or retirement. A predominate theme in geriatric communication involves the stress of living on a "fixed income." Social losses may occur through possible changes in prestige, status, and respect. Changes in sexual ability also may serve as a loss. The death of family members and friends creates additional interpersonal losses.(8)

Contemporaries may also be lost when friends migrate south for retirement.

Growing older may not always conform to the Robert Browning lines, "Grow old along with me! The best is yet to be." However, it need not be a time of frustration, pain, and helplessness. Most people fall within the middle range. Reactions to loss and change may vary from existential sadness to a temporary depressive response caused by a difficult day, an acute illness, a mourning reaction, to true clinical depression. Depression is often loosely defined. It "is a term applied to everything from transitory unhappiness to incapacitating suicidal despair."(9) However, because of the high incidence of depression in the elderly, we should be sensitive to this continuum and not just assume that feeling sad is a natural reaction to be expected in the elderly and therefore always dismiss depression as being just a normal consequence of aging.

> In clinical depression, the dysphoric mood (a feeling of discontent) lasts for at least 2 weeks and is accompanied by many symptoms: decreased energy; changes in appetite and weight; difficulty in sleep pattern; feelings of guilt, loneliness, hopelessness, helplessness, and worthlessness; somatic (bodily) complaints; difficulty in concentration and making decisions; crying easily; loss of sexual interest or pleasure; feeling everything is an effort; and recurrent thoughts of death or suicide.(8)

This syndrome is disabling in that it interferes with the patient's usual state of functioning.

A full range of mood disorders can affect the aged. The *Diagnostic and Statistical Manual of Mental Disorders* (DSM-III-R)(10) includes uncomplicated bereavement, adjustment disorder with depressed mood, depressive disorders (dysthymia, major depression), bipolar disorders (manic, depressed, and mixed types), and organic affective syndrome. Qualifiers include psychotic features, melancholic type, and seasonal pattern. We list these terms only to make you aware of the diagnostic challenge and intricacies of this diagnosis. It is beyond the confines of this book to elaborate further on these clinical syndromes.

Masked Depression. Another reason for underdiagnosis of depression in elderly people is the symptom variation that they often show. Masked depression is a common presentation in the geriatric patient. Here multiple, vague, nonspecific somatic (bodily) complaints in several body systems eclipse the dysphoric mood. "Depressive equivalents" include headache, chronic pain, gastrointestinal upsets (constipation, nausea), and decreased energy or drive. Other barometers of depression in elderly people include sleep disturbances or an internal feeling of nervousness or restlessness. Apathy with subtle ideation of failure, pessimism, loneliness, and hopelessness can be silent indications of underlying depression.(8)

Pseudodementia. Geriatric patients with major depression may present subjective complaints of deteriorating memory, difficulty in concentration, or difficulty in thinking. They may appear demented. If this cognitive impairment is reversible when the true depression is treated, the diagnosis is depression-induced organic mental disorder, or "pseudodementia." Jarik has noted that as many as one third of patients diagnosed as demented may suffer from depression.(11) "It is important to mention that a combination of depression with dementia in varying quantities is [also] a very frequent occurrence."(12)

Vignette: Marion and Tom

Marion and Tom had lived together for 33 years. During retirement they had been supportive of each other and had enjoyed their extra time together. Now Tom was getting deaf and slower in his movements. Marion was getting forgetful and finding it harder to care for their large Tudor home. The neighborhood was changing. It was definitely a time for change. Neither wanted to leave, as they saw their next move as their last. They were comfortable and secure in their family home. For some time, both stood firm against their son and daughter-in-law's suggestion that they move into an apartment in a retirement home. After spraining her ankle, which further limited her activities, Marion was the first to agree. Tom, however, grew withdrawn and depressed and threatened to live in the empty house alone. Their son reassured them and set firm limits. He rented a suitable apartment and told them that they would have to move by the end of summer. Three months later, they had made new friends in the building and were pleased with their new home.(1)

A Place to Live

"Aside from physical and emotional changes, housing and living arrangements present major concerns and bring to the fore florid misconceptions and often unrealistic expectations of this time of life. Many people believe that if they work hard and are good parents, they will be taken care of in their old age, but it does not always work out that way. 'Where shall we live?' can engender frustration and guilt and create problems of crisis proportions for all concerned."(1) Those adult children who are separated geographically may feel stressed trying to negotiate care long distance. Those who are near by may have mixed feelings about their role. The elderly are sometimes caught in the middle with their own set of thoughts and feelings. There are no easy or perfect solutions. The best rule of thumb is to plan ahead. Include the older person in the decision-making process and share your fears and concerns about the future.

"A popular myth about older people is that large numbers of them live in institutions of all kinds."(13) Although there are over a million nursing-home residents in the United States today, two-thirds of whom are women, only 5 percent of the older population will require such placement at any one time. No more than 20 to 30 percent of people over age 65 will ever have to spend time in a nursing home even for a short period of time.(14)

There are many housing alternatives for the elderly. The choice you make will depend on the medical and emotional needs of individuals as determined by their physicians as well as the reality of their available support network. These include allowing older persons to remain in their own homes, having them live with a relative, placing them in domiciliary care, or in a boarding home. Other options include residential care facilities (retirement homes) where the elderly will have room and at least one meal a day along with some social, recreational, and religious programs. A continuing care community will add additional personal and health care. If regular nursing, rehabilitative, and social services are required along with assistance with activities of daily living such as walking, dressing, eating, bathing, and the like, you may have to consider placement in an intermediate-care facility. If medical problems are more complex, requiring 24-hour medical care and supervision, a skilled nursing facility will be your choice. Each has its own pluses and minuses.

Their Home or Yours

Allowing the older person to remain in his or her own home or to live with a favorite relative may diminish the disorientation and need for change, which can precipitate symptoms of senility. However, this is not always the perfect answer. The elderly person living alone may neglect his or her nutritional and emotional needs until much harm has been done. Husbands and wives, brothers and sisters, or other couples living together can become so set in their ways that they often support each other's distrust and reluctance to allow outside help into the home (a *folie à deux*). When an older person moves in with his or her son or daughter, a new set of problems can develop. Old, unresolved conflicts between parents and other siblings often come to the fore. The older person may even find himself or herself the focus of a family fight. Environmental change often required during the later years can be fraught with resistance and unknown complications.(1)

If you do decide to keep an older person at home, community services are available. Don't feel that you have to do everything yourself. A home health care nursing agency can provide homemaker or home health aid services. Nursing personnel and social workers, as well as physical, occupational, and speech therapists, offer in-home services. Home-delivered meals, visitor programs, transportation, and escort services are available. Senior programs can provide lunch as well as activities and socialization for the ambulatory, higher functioning elderly. Adult day programs can provide social and health care services and provide temporary relief for caregivers. The National Support Center for Families of the Aging in Swarthmore, Pennsylvania, provides a newsletter and other educational information.

Choosing the right placement for your aging parents is not easy. The main variable must be a realistic assessment of their medical needs. You cannot make them young again. In that you may be wearing emotional blinders, it is often best to rely on the health care team, including physician, psychiatrist, nursing personnel, social worker, and physical therapist, to assess the level of care that is needed. Another important variable will be your own needs and family situation. You may have to accept that you cannot fill all the physical and emotional needs of your older relatives. Although you may go to great lengths to keep your loved ones at home, you may find that their care requirements are beyond your means or ability. This will be the time to choose another option such as nursing home placement.

Nursing Home Placement

It is helpful to begin the search for a housing alternative long before it is really needed. The admission process may be complex. No vacancies and long waiting lists are not uncommon. I often counsel families to do their homework and place their loved one on the waiting list before a crisis precipitates the search for solutions. This way, they avoid the stress of placement in an emergency situation. Obtain a list of homes in your area from the phone book, state and local community agencies, the social service department of your hospital, or a senior program. Begin the process of elimination by calling and visiting the facilities, armed with questions about services, activities, and finances. Legal arrangements may have to be made in reference to personal funds and options for the future. Decisions will have to be made concerning personal belongings. Some will have to be sold or given away. Bringing some objects along will help make the new home more familiar and attractive.

Deciding to place a parent in a nursing home can be an extremely stressful time, showing a complex interplay between generations. Feelings will be intense. The adult child must deal with feelings of guilt and come to grips with the expectation that if she truly loved her parent, she would take care of the parent at home. Many call to ask my advice. I usually tell them that if the parent or older relative requires more care or structure than it is possible for them to give at home, then the loved one should be placed in a nursing home.

It is also important to think of yourself in this situation. It is not selfishness but rather self-survival. The parent, on the other hand, may be fearful that the home will not really be a home. He or she may feel that it is the last stop before death—the beginning of the end—or may also have angry feelings: "I looked after my spouse and now there is no one to look after me." All involved will feel sad and suffer a sense of grieving for something that will be no longer. "We won't be able to go to grandma's house any more."

Both parent and adult child need to see that placement may really be a new beginning, that a nursing home can be a place where the parent will be well cared for. Intermediate and skilled nursing facilities can provide a pleasant setting for the geriatric patient who requires that level of medical care. In such a place, they receive medication and specialized therapy, such as physical therapy and occupational therapy, and will not be an undue burden to their families. Such facilities provide more structure than is possible in the home setting, a perfect arrangement for the more dependent individual. A good nursing home can provide stimulation through exercise therapy, entertainment, and recreation. In some cases, it can be a setting where the elderly can potentially make new friends. Many tap the resources of the community and volunteers.

Try to choose a home that is near those people who will be visiting most frequently. Visitors are very important in maintaining the patient's morale and emotional well being. The presence of family members and friends helps create a more personal atmosphere and reassurance occurs that someone still cares. Aside from the company, nursing home residents enjoy and appreciate little gifts of favorite foods (check dietary restrictions) that may not be available in the home. Where needed, nursing home personnel will appreciate family members who can aid with personal care services such as feeding, dressing, and exercise. Visitors may be allowed to supplement the resident's activity choices by taking them outside or on short trips into the community.

On the negative side, although the need for nursing home care is escalating, the number of trained nursing home personnel is not. Many nursing home patients have mental health problems such as dementia and depression. Others show behavioral problems such as agitation and verbal and physical abusiveness. Noisy, wandering, and combative patients can easily wear down staff. Such difficult behavior can also take away staff time from other patients.(15) At their worst, nursing homes can be ill-smelling warehouses in which the older person is dehumanized, may lose his or her sense of autonomy, and can be at the mercy of overworked and intolerant personnel. You will need to choose your facility with care. A nursing home ombudsman is available through the state or local office on aging to help if you experience problems in a nursing home. The ombudsman can investigate complaints and instigate corrective action. Flyers indicating their services are usually posted on bulletin boards on each floor of a nursing facility.

Legal and Ethical Dilemmas

If you are involved with the care of an elderly person in the 1990s, you will be involved with several complex ethical issues and will need to have some understanding of certain legal matters. The following are meant simply to prompt your awareness. For more detailed information consult your attorney. Plan ahead. Talk to your parents about their finances and their choices. Get information about the location of wills, deeds, stock certificates, cemetery lot deeds, and other legal papers. There are several things they can do before they are disabled and while they are still legally competent.

Make a will. Persons can make a will if they know, without prompting, that they are doing so, the names and their relationship to the people who will receive their property, and the nature and extent of the property.(16)

Sign a power of attorney. This document gives another person authority to manage your affairs and act in your behalf. It can be limited to specific duties such as paying bills or selling a house, or may give broader powers. Regular powers of attorney are no longer valid if the person becomes incompetent. Under these circumstances, a durable power of attorney allows the surrogate's power of decision to continue. Every state and the District of Columbia has adopted general durable power of attorney statutes.

Make a living will. A living will is a written document that specifies the circumstances under which a person will permit the cessation of extraordinary treatment to prolong life, and would allow death in accordance with the natural progression of their disease.(17) For instance, it may indicate that in the event of terminal illness, when the person is incapable of participating in medical decisions, no life-sustaining measures used merely to postpone the moment of death, be used. Not every state recognizes the legality of the living will.

Guardianship

If a person is no longer competent, that is, he or she is not able to understand what treatment, procedure, or placement is being proposed and is unable to manage his or her affairs and/or property effectively, you may become involved in a guardianship of property or of the person procedure. If involuntary hospitalization for psychiatric treatment is needed, you will have to petition for a *conservatorship.* In these procedures, an attorney files a petition in court and a hearing before a judge takes place. The patient's physician and/or a psychiatrist may be asked to supply a medical report and/or expert testimony. The judge will decide if the person is legally competent. He may then appoint a legal guardian to act for the person in financial matters, order the needed care, or send the person to a hospital.

Do Not Resuscitate Decisions (DNR)

When hospitalized, a DNR or "no code" decision may have to be made. This is a request that no extraordinary or heroic measures be initiated in the event that the patient stops breathing or their heart stops. If a DNR order is given and documented, no active therapy, such as initiation of mechanical life support devices (for example, artificial ventilation and/or emergency cardiopulmonary resuscitation), will be used. Conservative passive medical care will be given to promote the patient's well-being and relieve suffering. The patient can make this decision if he or she is competent and capable of making an informed decision consent. If not, the legal next-of-kin or legal guardian can make this decision. Advanced directives, such as durable powers of attorney and living wills, need to be taken into account where they exist. One may request CPR but refuse an artificial breathing machine or vice versa. DNR orders may be cancelled verbally at any time by a capable patient or surrogate.

The Caregiver Role

People now live longer. In time, the emotional and physical dependence of your aging parents will increase. You will gradually experience a subtle shift in the balance of power. Roles will reverse and you will become your parents' parents. Often this is a difficult role to accept. As Mom and Dad become older and less able to care for themselves, you will also enter a difficult, painful, and confusing stage of life. To be confronted with some of the problems of aging can be frightening just when you are starting to notice that you are getting older and have started to face your own mortality. There will be genuine sorrow and a deep sense of loss as you see those mighty figures of your childhood becoming more needy and vulnerable.

Adult children can face enormous pressures as they become the major support system for their aging parents. The emotional toll is heavy. As a caregiver, you will feel concerned, compassionate, worried, and responsible. As they become more disabled, their social and financial dependence on you will increase. You will give your time and money and moral support. You will want to help with their needs but may also sometimes feel trapped, overburdened, and angry. Other emotional reactions include feelings of helplessness, embarrassment, guilt, resentfulness, and confusion. You may even be filled with self-pity. You will be upset and frustrated when they do not take your advice or accept your offers to help. You will struggle with fatigue, depression, and isolation.(18,19)

Becoming a caregiver to a chronically ill aging relative is a gesture of love. Many show a fierce determination to keep their parent or other relative at home. Taking care of an elderly parent is similar in some ways to taking care of children. However, regardless of the degree of mental impairment, the elderly person's basic personality is still intact and you will need to treat him or her as an adult, not a child. Unlike children, aging parents come complete with a history and set of personality traits that can become even more accentuated with age and stress. Include them in any decision-making process. Expect older persons to fulfill responsibilities in the house up to their limitations. Encourage them to maintain socially acceptable behavior including personal hygiene, clothing, and manners. Encourage them to do for themselves as much as possible. Taking over all aspects of their life may not be necessary and can undermine confidence and self-esteem.

An important role for the caregiver is to serve as a source of reality testing for the elderly. Be sure a clock, calendar, bulletin board for schedules, and specific placement of frequently used items are available to jog their memory. Encourage them to read the newspaper and watch the news on television. Try to discuss current events with them. Respond to confusion with facts. Allow the older person to be involved in the life of the family. Express your positive feelings. Tell them you care. Touch can be a healing gesture. Love, affection, attention, and nurturing from family members, including grandchildren, can do wonders to improve moody dispositions and negative behavior. Older people appreciate compliments also. Pets and plants in the environment can also be helpful as they provide stimulation and reduce self-centeredness by encouraging them to invest in something outside of themselves.

Encourage your parents to share their history and experiences. The life review can be therapeutic for them and rewarding for you and your children. Have them tell you their tales of the past; their joys and sorrows, defeats and triumphs. You will come to recognize and appreciate the uniqueness of their lives. Early photographs can be used to aid memory and stimulate emotions. In gaining a better perspective of the forces that influenced their lives, both you and your children may emerge with a better understanding and appreciation of your roots and identity and some of the background that influenced your own personality.(20)

Avoiding Stress and Burnout

Burnout occurs when unrealistically high expectations cause you to experience emotional and physical fatigue. The need to provide constant care for an elderly individual can be a strain. You will know you are there when you find you are more irritable than usual, feeling moody and depressed, arguing more with your spouse, family members, or co-workers, or reaching for a pill or alcoholic beverage to solve the problem. You may have vague physical complaints, begin losing weight, and have difficulty sleeping. A difficult situation can cause a failure of coping mechanisms in even a normal personality, particularly if you feel trapped, frustrated, and fatigued. (See Chapter 8 for additional information on stress.)

The following are some of the things you can do to combat caregiver burnout:

Have realistic expectations. Don't try to be super caregiver. There are no magic solutions. Try for a balance between the ideal and reality. You can provide for the needs of your aging parents but cannot solve all of their problems. You cannot make them young again. You cannot make them happy or be responsible for their happiness. Sometimes just listening is enough; you do not always have to do something. Perhaps they are just ventilating frustration. Have reasonable expectations about your own behavior. Don't expect yourself to always be cheerful. Feeling irritable is often part of the caregiver persona.

Make use of support systems. There is help available in the community, including homemaker services and counseling, which you can make use of before problems become overwhelming. There are resources to provide transportation to the doctor, meals, and recreational activities. Adult day care can allow you to take a break. Your county council on aging can provide more information. The caregiver also needs support. Don't hold in your feelings. Talk it out and share your emotions with family and friends. Children-of-senior-parents support groups can be helpful for the adult child caregiver. They will show you that you are not alone and are not a terrible person. Here you can share your feelings as well as trade advice and information.

Plan ahead. Constructive worrying is helpful. Plan what to do if things go wrong. Investigate and instigate nursing home or other institutional placement before a crisis occurs. Don't avoid discussing such issues as health insurance, finances, wills, burial arrangements, and their views on life support or living wills.

Ask for help. It is not uncommon for one family member to take primary care of a parent regardless of the number of other available relatives. If you are to be effective in caring for your aging parent, you must have occasional relief. Sometimes family members will not volunteer because they know that you will do it. Ask your brothers and sisters for help. You may be able to divide up chores or take turns providing care. Ask them to share in the cost of caring for your parent. Try to be assertive rather than aggressive and demanding. Neighbors, friends, and other interested parties in the community can also be called on to provide you with help.

Guidelines for Caregiver Success

- *Do it voluntarily.* There are no laws that require you to provide physical care for the elderly. Take on the role because you want to and not because you feel you have to out of obligation, guilt, or even love. Doing so will give you a greater sense of control, prevent you from feeling trapped, and help you be a caregiver in a way that best fits your own situation. You are allowed to write your own job description. Expectations are not binding unless you put them into effect. Becoming a caregiver is really a choice regardless of your motivations. If you can see caregiving as a voluntary choice, you are more apt to be successful in the role.
- *Resolve old feelings.* To work with the elderly you have to be free of old baggage. You have to have resolved your feelings about your parents or grandparents as well as your feelings about growing older. If you still feel that old people should be obeyed and feared, then you will have difficulty. You will also be ineffective if you are threatened by old age or overidentify with their feelings of loneliness, depression, or fearfulness. The older person in your house may not be the same as the parent you remember. You may be frustrated if you expect to start where you left off many years before. They may no longer have the capacity to resolve old issues or interact in the

way you expect. You may have to get to know a very different person.

- *Be good to yourself.* Don't neglect the quality of your life. Don't isolate yourself. Take time for yourself. Make use of as many techniques as you can to relax and rest. Exercise to work off aggressive energy. Leave time for relaxation (a decompression zone) between work and home. Lighten the situation with laughter. You may need some privacy and time for yourself. Get away from it all at times by scheduling a long weekend or other time off. Take care of yourself. Your emotional and physical health is also important.

- *Know your limits.* Set limits on how much you are able to do and give. Present it in a positive way. Don't compromise out of love or guilt. Step back and see if your parent is demanding too much or if you are asking too much of yourself. It is all right to take your own needs into account when deciding on care for an elderly parent.

- *Don't neglect the others in your household.* This includes your spouse and adolescent children. The problems involved in three generations living together can be great. No matter how hard you try, the emotional equilibrium in your family relationships will change once you bring an elderly relative into your house. This can lead to conflicts and misunderstandings. Being a caregiver can also affect the balance of your marriage as new responsibilities leave you less time to interact with your spouse. Schedule time to be together. Fatigue can start to erode your sexual desire. Frustration and irritability can land on those you love most. You will have to continue to work on these important relationships. Don't expect your spouse to feel exactly the same way as you do. Good communication will help and can also increase the emotional bond between you.

- *Communicate openly.* Good communication between all family members in the household is one of the most important aspects of coping successfully with an impaired elderly person in your home. A family conference or meeting, with or without the help of a counselor, can be helpful in resolving problems and making plans. The key to good communication is nonjudgmental active listening where you accept each others' feelings. Keep communication open and honest with your parents also. Tell them how you feel and include them in any decision-making process.

- *Try not to feel guilty.* Caregivers are already carrying a heavy burden. They do not need to be further weighed down with guilt. Don't feel guilty about your feelings. Resentment, angry feelings, and even an occasional death wish does not mean you are a bad person or hate your parent. Such thoughts may only mean that you are under stress. Sometimes you may promise or want to do more than is possible. This is human. You may feel that you are in a no-win situation torn between your life and the life of your parent. Don't feel guilty about taking care of your own needs. This is not being selfish; it is self-preservation.

Remember, there is no one "right way" to provide care for an elderly parent or relative.

Death with Dignity

We all tend to live as if we had unlimited time. However, death is universal. All living organisms die. Man has always wrestled with the enigma of death. All of us must work out our own answer to the meaning of life and death. The scientific and intellectual reality is that death is the end of life—the cessation of all physical and mental functioning. Emotionally, dying is the final phase of life.

In the United States, we tend to have few rituals that prepare us for death. However, each person is unique and this uniqueness needs to be respected as the individual approaches death. People tend to die as they have lived. They should be able to utilize their remaining time according to their own priorities. Some will want to make detailed funeral arrangements, take care of practical and psychological unfinished business, or give away valued possessions. During this time inner psychic shifts will occur which need to be respected. Their sense of time may be changed. You will have to be available when they feel the need rather than asking them to adjust to you.(21)

There is much debate as to whether to tell a terminally ill patient that they are dying. Perhaps the question should really be how to tell them rather than whether they should be told. People have a tendency to tune out what they do not want to deal with. In order to help your dying parent, you must be able to deal with the reality of death yourself. (See Chapter 10 for additional information about coping with the death of a parent.) Many times people avoid the dying patient because they are afraid of dealing with this inevitable reality and/or cannot tolerate the feeling of helplessness that this confrontation can elicit.

In truth, this final time at the end of the line is important for the dying person and their family members. It can be a time for both sides to express positive feelings which have been unspoken. It is a time when your parent may wish to make specific decisions and set his or her house in order. It is a time when you can help them die with peace and dignity by maintaining a sense of hopefulness, answering their questions honestly, allowing them to express their feelings, being sure that they are free of pain, and being there so that they will not die alone. Thus you may mourn but you will not have regrets. No one can ever take away your fond memories of your loved one. Their light will continue to shine on you.

Chapter 13

Middle-Aged Wisdom

What a man knows at 50 that he did not at 20 is, for the most part, incommunicable. The laws, the aphorisms, the generalizations, the universal truths, the parables, and the old saws—all of the observations about life which can be communicated handily in ready, verbal packages—are as well known to a man at 20 who has been attentive as to a man at 50. He has been told them all, he has read them all, and he has probably repeated them all before he graduates from college; but he has not lived them all.

What he knows at 50 that he did not know at 20 boils down to something like this: The knowledge he has acquired with age is not the knowledge of formulas, or forms of words, but of people, places, actions—a knowledge not gained by words but by touch, sight, sound, victories, failures, sleeplessness, devotion, love— the human experiences and emotions of this earth and of oneself and of other men; and perhaps, too, a little faith, and a little reverence for things you cannot see.

ADLAI STEVENSON
1954 Graduation Speech
Princeton University

Stevenson was right. What changes in middle age is not what we actually know, but the shading and nuances that give new meaning to things. What changes is perspective. You gain an ability to see the whole picture. A new clarity develops about what is really important in life. You gain a new appreciation of good health, with freedom from emotional and physical pain,

211

and meaningful relationships which lingers long after the material goals are reached and the money is spent. The developmental crisis of midlife begins with the loss of youth but ends with the acquisition of a few gray hairs, some wisdom, more self-confidence, and the power that comes with the authority of experience. When you were young, you felt that you knew it all. It is only later that you realize just how long it takes to gain real maturity.

Middle age is like being in a prizefight with life. Anxiety and tension can be high. You may get bruised and knocked about a bit, but most people eventually win the bout. You come out of the ring with a heightened sense of fulfillment, contentment, and understanding. You spend a little more time taking care of yourself, enjoying the simpler pleasures, and paying attention to the quality of your life. Perhaps you even remember to kiss your children and grandchildren more often, say thank you and show more appreciation for some of the simple things in life, and are a bit kinder to the people you meet along the way. Somehow you become more tolerant. A grandmother tells me, "My daughter gets so frustrated with the children. I try to tell her that they are just being kids."

We take so much for granted, particularly relationships and our health. In middle life, things can happen that make us suddenly aware of what we had. An illness or accident comes out of the blue, divorce occurs, a child is hurt, a friend or parent dies, and in hindsight we wish we had been different, shifted our emphasis somewhat, and paid more attention to relationships and the small wonders of life. Sometimes we realize too late that we could have taken better care of ourselves or spent more time with or actually said the words "I love you" to a cherished relative or friend.

Rabbi Harold Kushner summed it up well in his book *When All You Ever Wanted Isn't Enough*.(1) He advises middle-aged persons who are looking for life's meaning and are unhappy because they feel that something is missing in their lives to stop searching for the great answer and "learn to savor the moment, even if it does not last forever." He says that middle age "is a time to 'eat our bread in gladness and drink our wine in joy' not despite the fact that life does not go on forever but precisely because of that fact. It is a time to enjoy happiness with those we love and to realize that we are at a time in our lives when enjoying today means more than worrying about tomorrow. It is a time to celebrate that fact that we have finally learned what life is about and how to make the most of it." Such are the insights and revelations of middle age.

Why Didn't Someone Tell Me?

Life isn't always easy. It can be chaotic and unpredictable. As we go through the life cycle, we become more aware of our vulnerability, our mortality, and our lack of control over people and many of the things that happen to us. Middle age may be the first time we have to face these realities. In over 20 years of practicing clinical psychiatry, I have seen many patients forlorn and depressed, angry and resentful about where the train of life has brought them. Many lament, "Why didn't someone tell me? I thought it would be different." Whether the presenting problem is adolescent turmoil, marital conflict, menopause and midlife crises, dealing with illness or physical pain, or adjusting to growing older, the confusion and disillusionment is often the same. Middle age, as well as the other stages of life, can be frustrating if we do not temper our expectations, have a clear understanding of the age-specific problems that may be met along the way, find some possible solutions, and acquire coping skills.

In the general practice of psychiatry, we often have to help people come to grips with the realities of life, correct misconceptions, and gain a new insightful perspective. We aren't trained to be parents or caregivers. We soon learn that life doesn't always follow the fairy-tale version we imagined as a child. We have to work at relationships. We have to be assertive and find our own way. Whether the complaint is marital, occupational, or interpersonal, a certain acceptance of the human condition is necessary to make progress. Perfection must be seen as only wishful thinking. Reality must replace fantasy. We are really alone and responsible for our own actions and decisions. We must push forward in a problem-solving manner. There is often more than one correct and possible solution to a problem. Neither problem solving nor life is ever black or white. Shades of gray need to become our favorite color.

Many people come for therapy because they find that their life experiences have not fulfilled their expectations or fantasies. Perplexed and angry, they may be showing clinical evidence of anxiety, depression, or one of the other psychiatric syndromes we have reviewed in earlier chapters. However, regardless of specific diagnosis, they all have misconceptions, lack of information, and obstructive ways of communicating their basic needs. During the course of individual or group psychotherapy, I find myself over and over again trying to explain the same themes, correct the same misconceptions, and give the same perspectives. I have dealt with many of these issues in this book. Hopefully, you will have gained new insights in reading its pages and become more adept at solving your conflicts and sense of unhappiness. Yes, life can be full of trials and tribulations but it can also be fulfilling and good. Armed with these new insights, you can no longer say, "Why didn't someone tell me? I thought it would be different."

Therapy: Is It Really the Answer?

People often fear psychiatrists and psychotherapy. This is a shame. Regardless of their level of education, some individuals feel that therapists can read their minds. Many are embarrassed and ashamed to talk about events in their lives because they feel that they will be seen as "bad," sinful, or unusual. People routinely believe that what has happened to them is unique and therefore will be criticized, not understood, and certainly not accepted. Most of what I hear in therapy, I have heard before. People's lives are not really that unique. Patients feel that they will have to give up control in therapy. Many think they will lose their jobs or the respect of their friends and family if they seek psychiatric help. Some feel they will be declared "crazy" and shuttled off to a mental institution. Such unfounded beliefs stop many from getting much-needed help. Nothing strange or unusual happens in therapy. Guided by the psychiatrist, we simply talk to one another.

Technically,

> a psychiatrist is a physician whose specialty is the diagnosis and treatment of people suffering from mental disorders. . . . [He or she] can provide a comprehensive evaluation from a psychiatric point of view, a medical differential diagnosis, treatment planning and multiple therapeutic and health-enhancing interventions. The psychiatrist can then integrate this historical and examination material with the physical . . . and laboratory findings relevant to the symptoms [presented] . . . to evolve a diagnostic system [medical differential diagnosis] from which the treatment and discharge plans . . . are produced. Treatment methods may include biological, somatic, and interpersonal interventions including all of the forms of psychotherapy and psychoeducation and the skilled combination of these. It is this capacity to integrate all of these medical findings, and to use whatever treatment interventions are necessary and appropriate to influence them positively, that makes the psychiatrist unique.(2)

However, the therapeutic relationship can offer so much more. It can truly be a healing relationship. It is important to make a commitment to therapy based on facts and to find a therapist with whom you feel comfortable. Psychiatrists are physicians and human beings. They should not be placed on a pedestal. Some are good and some are mediocre. You may have to shop around until you find a therapist with whom you can genuinely open up and talk. At the end of a first office evaluation, I will usually try to see if I understand where the patient is emotionally and what has happened to him or her to bring them to this point in his or her life. After sharing my brief formulation, I usually ask patients three questions. I want to know if they feel reasonably comfortable talking to me, if what I have said to them makes sense, and if they felt that I was truly talking about them in my remarks. If we can both answer yes to these questions, then at least we know that we have made a start and can go forward in therapy.

Ask your family physician or referral source for the names of two or three possible therapists. Talk to them on the phone or in person. Be sure to ask about their training and therapeutic perspective. Psychotherapeutic intervention can run the gamut from the psychoanalytic to behavioral to supportive. Although trained in psychoanalytically oriented psychotherapy, I myself prefer an eclectic approach. In doing individual medical psychotherapy and group psychotherapy, I try to make use of whatever methods I can to help the patient. Spend time finding the therapist that seems right for you and with whom you feel comfortable. Once rapport and trust have been established, many wonderful things can happen.

In this book, we have reviewed some of the normal stresses of daily life that can occur during middle age. We have also given you information on some of the mental health problems that can occur from adolescence to old age. We have tried to educate you so that you could gain a more realistic perspective. Hopefully, if one of these problems happens in your life to yourself or someone you love, you will be better able to cope with these events. Many of the problems of living that were mentioned, as well as all of the more specific mental health syndromes that were described, could benefit from talking to a knowledgeable but objective individual such as a psychiatrist. The doctor–patient relationship is a powerful therapeutic force capable of producing many positive changes. In an atmosphere of acceptance, empathy, and neutrality, the psychotherapist actively listens, asks questions, provides information, reassurance, and perspective, orders medication when necessary, and helps you start to understand yourself and your world.

In a supportive, nonjudgmental milieu, the psychotherapist can help you relax and express painful feelings and prior traumas. He or she can take you seriously and try to understand the meaning particular stressful or traumatic events had for you. The therapist can give positive feedback. Therapy can reduce guilt feelings. It can help place things in perspective, suggest alternatives, and provide a degree of reality testing by acting not so much as the echo of conscience but as the quiet voice of reason. The psychotherapist can provide a nurturing atmosphere conducive to change and growth. Slowly, he or she can move you along the road toward maturity and the acceptance of life. Unfortunately, many who have received help in therapy keep it a secret because of the stigma of having been a psychiatric patient. Thus others, unaware of the positive aspects of psychotherapy, are prevented from seeking help until it is an emergency.

Don't Be Afraid of the Dark

People seem to be more afraid of their mind and its workings than their physical functioning. Perhaps this is because feelings and the symptoms of mental illness represent more of an unknown and still carry much of a stigma. I asked a patient of mine, who was suffering from anxiety symptoms, her ideas on this subject. "Being lightheaded and anxious is the worst thing in the world. It's horrifying. You're not in control of yourself." She said that she could point to, touch, and conceptualize physical pain and discomfort. Therefore, they were not as frightening or as much of an unknown as were emotional symptoms. It seems to be the added dimension of feeling out of control that routinely comes across as the main reason why patients fear emotional symptoms and feel that they are worse than physical symptoms.

Another patient adds, "It's easier to take care of physical symptoms. If you break an arm, you go and get it fixed. It's hard to change your personality." People also feel that a heart attack or other physical ill is unpredictable and out of their control. However, they feel that they "should" be able to control their emotions and are therefore harder on themselves and also feel more out of control when they have emotional problems. To many, the mind is a dark unknown area that is frightening and beyond their control.

Although the relationship between mind and body has been debated by philosophers such as Leibnitz, Descartes, and Hobbes throughout the history of thought, an insistence on this strict dichotomy is less logical in the 1990s than ever before. The predominant theoretical framework in psychiatry and medical science today is the biopsychosocial model, which suggests that the mind and body act on each other in remarkable ways. This systems theory says that nature is arranged in a hierarchical continuum, where nothing exists in isolation and all levels of organization are linked and influence one another. The identity of a system as a whole (for example, a person), including its properties and functioning, emerge out of the dynamic interaction of the components that make up the system. Mental phenomena, therefore, are different from but do emerge from the physiological and physicochemical events of brain processing in the nervous system.(3)

The extraordinary interrelationship between biological and psychosocial factors is becoming clearer. It has been shown, for instance, that emotions can affect the immune system because the two are joined by a hormonal, chemical, "feedback loop."(4) Brain neurophysiology clearly influences emotional symptoms. For example, a brain abnormality has been identified that makes one more vulnerable to panic attacks.(5) It is now felt that "panic disorder is a result of specific stressful life events, most commonly separation or loss, in a person with a specific biologic (genetic or acquired) vulnerability."(6)

Don't be afraid of your mind. Don't be afraid of the unknown. Don't be afraid of the dark. The mind really is understandable and more predictable than you think. The unknown can be positive. Knowledge, understanding, and perspective gained in therapy can do much to lift the veil of darkness. As you better understand yourself and your mind, you will be less fearful. You may start acting differently and others may respond differently to you. Things can change. Something positive can happen. One thing leads to another. The confidence and increased self-esteem that you can gain in therapy, along with the increased energy which is no longer bound up in worry, depression, and anxiety, can do much to free you and propel you in new, more positive directions.

Emotional symptoms and behavior have meaning and may serve a restorative function. They may be a sign that you are trying to cope with things that are happening inside and outside of yourself. They may be an attempt to deal with feelings such as anxiety, anger, or inadequacy. For instance, persons who are extremely angry at someone and cannot deal with these feelings may become paranoid, projecting their negative feelings to another and then believing that the other person is against them or trying to harm them. As we saw in Chapter 4, even substance abuse can be a means of adapting and a symptom reflecting some sort of psychological stress. It may be the only mechanism the person has available to cope with problems of living and try to master some form of personal imbalance, conflict, or excitation.(7)

As we have seen, even the midlife crisis can be a sign that the individual is trying to cope with internal and external changes and pressures. Confronted with the discrepancy between what they thought life would be and how it actually turned out, they try to reconcile personal, relationship, and occupational goals. Trying to adjust to health changes, face their own mortality, handle the loss of children who are moving on their own, and cope with the trials and tribulations of aging parents, they often run in different directions before finding a happy medium.

Generations: What Do They Want from Each Other?

In over 20 years of practicing clinical psychiatry, I have learned a great deal about what people want and need. People share much in common. Strip away the material and educational differences and erase the competition, the jealousies, and the anger, and you will find a human being behind the facade and the mask who is just trying to make it through. People do differ in their ability to be empathetic, their degree of sensitivity, and their ability to feel guilt and remorse. They differ in their coping mechanisms. However, underneath it all, they share similar emotions and needs. Each generation has its own jargon, customs, and social patterns. However, the trials and tribulations of life and the accompanying feelings are the same. Men and women, parents and children are all vulnerable, can be hurt, and feel emotional and physical pain.

Many times in therapy, patients complain that their parents, children, spouses, and friends are not fulfilling their needs. They seem to be asking for love, attention, acknowledgment, and understanding. They want to be treated with respect and dignity. They want to feel needed and not be taken for granted. They respond to kindness and empathy and a caring attitude. They blossom and grow and show increased self-esteem if they are complimented. They require trust and a feeling of security. They want relief from feelings of guilt and validation that they are not bad people. They need laughter to help reduce tension and not take themselves so seriously. They want to know that they are not crazy and perhaps not as emotionally ill as they thought. Often they need reassurance that they will not die, lose control, or go crazy. They want to be free of pain.

People show different degrees of emotional and behavioral maturity. Many are responsible and can take care of themselves. They can do the various chores that life requires to survive but have much difficulty sharing feelings. A very simplistic way to judge a person's level of emotional maturity is to see how they communicate and accept feelings of love and anger. Can they say, I love you? Can they accept it if someone gives them a compliment or says they care? People often feel that if they express feelings of love, they will be vulnerable and can be hurt. They therefore hold back on the three words that can open the door to happiness, intimacy, and positive feedback. For some, it is hard to say "I love you."

It is equally important to be able to tell someone that you are upset with their behavior and have the ability to accept criticism and negative feelings without feeling that you are totally bad. People often worry that sharing negative feelings will drive people away or hurt them. They worry about telling people how they feel. Tell people your feelings. Often it can lead to increased understanding and closeness. In therapy, we often encourage people to share their feelings, but mix it with kindness if it is something that they do not want to hear. Tell them the positive along with the negative. It is equally important, at times, to be diplomatic and not bombard people in your life with your feelings. Hold back if the other person truly cannot handle the information. It works both ways. Be kind to one another.

Each generation, from adolescence to the elderly, wants the same things. They all have basic physiologic needs for nourishment and rest. However, they also have other needs. These include the following:

Love, affection, and tenderness. These are needed and appreciated at every age. Sex is part of this equation but so is physical touch, a kind word, and companionship. We all need comforting and nurturing at times. We need to know that someone cares. Praise can help a person to blossom.

Acceptance and approval. All people want to be accepted for who they are—warts and all. Being a whole person includes the positive and the negative. Children of all ages need this type of recognition from their parents. It can foster a positive relationship that will be helpful in all future relationships including marriage, child rearing, and career.

Intimacy. Being close to another human being with whom you can share your secrets and your life can add another dimension to existence. Intimacy is a basic human need. We all need to love and be loved.

Honesty and trust. According to Thomas Jefferson, honesty is the first chapter of the book of wisdom. Trust provides a sense of security. Good communication in therapy or life can be a buffer against stress. Patients often worry about what to tell people about what has happened in their lives. "My son got divorced; my husband lost his job; my child died." Filled with shame, grief, hurt, or anger, they ask, "What should I tell them?" The answer is simple; hit them with reality. The easiest answer is to be straightforward and tell them the simple truth without elaboration.

Hope. A psychotic patient of mine, now in remission, told me that she had read a best-seller about mental illness. She said that the one thing she got out of the book was hope. "The story told me that you can get better from a mental illness." The late Norman Cousins, author of the book *Anatomy of an Illness*, was a strong believer that hope is a potent weapon against disease and a vital ingredient in healing even serious illness.

Respect and dignity. We all want to maintain our self-esteem, be taken seriously, and be treated with consideration. This is particularly relevant with the elderly as they face failing health, social, and emotional losses.

Freedom from pain. Emotional and physical pain are part of life at times. We have to be thankful if they are not a part of our lives. Life is not always fair. It is not always true that if we do everything right that everything will turn out just fine. Bad things do happen to good people. The world is sometimes chaotic and unpredictable. However, as the poet John Dryden said, "sweet is pleasure after pain."(8) Sometimes, freedom from pain allows us to appreciate the pleasures that we have and be more empathetic of the trials and tribulations of our fellow human beings.

Guidelines for Success

- *Be active.* The key to a successful life is to stay involved and maintain a passion for work and other projects. Strive toward a goal and don't ever be without one. Continue to learn and grow. We all need something to look forward to, something to wake up for. Be creative and remain productive. Invest yourself in others. These characteristics can do much to add satisfaction and fulfillment to your life. It can also lead to generativity as you share your knowledge and mentor younger people.
- *Take risks.* We are not talking about impulsive behavior here but rather actions calculated on information and education. Many, for instance, may stay in a boring job for years, fearful to change and yet too insecure to take a risk. They seem to assume that change will always be negative; however, change often brings positive results. Try different things. Take a risk and do something new.
- *Pay attention to relationships.* You must consciously and consistently work on relationships that are important to you. They must be lovingly nurtured and not taken for granted. Adolescent turmoil may cause fireworks; later we may wonder what all the heat was about. Family members and others are not perfect. Sometimes it is best not to take their words or behavior at face value. Don't close the door on relationships with those you love. Each interaction can be a new beginning. In the long run, it is these emotional bonds we form with parents, children, and friends that sustain us and provide quality in our lives.
- *Accept others as they are.* Interpersonal relationships are not always easy. You cannot change other people. You can only take responsibility for your own actions and your half of the interaction. We are all human with good and bad points. If you expect everyone to be perfect you

will constantly be frustrated. Have realistic expectations of others.

- *Take care of yourself.* Have your own life. Don't just rely on others to make you happy. Pay attention to the quality of your life. Develop interests and friendships that are meaningful to you. Take care of your body. Pay attention to nutrition and rest. It is all right to slow down a little. Leave time for relaxation and fun. Get medical treatment early before physical problems escalate.
- *Take an assertive problem-solving approach to life.* Use your energy for growth rather than the neurotic pursuit of trying to change that which can not be changed. Commitment is important to success in interpersonal relationships and other life endeavors.

  1. Evaluate your needs and expectations.
  2. Decide what you want.
  3. Make a commitment to it.
  4. Work at making it a reality.

- *Ask for what you want.* Pride and fear of rejection often stand in the way. Asking for what you want is important in both your personal and business life. In business, particularly, you don't always get what you deserve; you get what you negotiate and communicate. It is not a guarantee of success but people cannot read your mind. Do not assume that everyone thinks the same way. They all have been brought up by different parents and raised in a different emotional environment. Verbalize your feelings, concerns, and needs.
- *Have realistic expectations of yourself.* In this book we have shared much information about middle-aged experiences and what can happen to people from adolescence through old age. We hope that it will be helpful. However, remember, information and understanding can be useful but they do not guarantee success. They alone will not make you a perfect parent or child. There are many things

that are not under our control. Allow yourself to be human. Children, for instance, usually give their parents higher marks on parenting than they might give themselves. Make peace with who you are and believe in yourself. Accept your limitations.

- *Maintain a support network.* Even independent people need someone to lean on at times for emotional security. One person may not be able to fulfill all of your needs. Isolation is not helpful to good mental health. Involvement with others can reduce feelings of depression and increase confidence and self-esteem. Independent people often do not like to talk about their dependency needs and will feel more comfortable using the phrase "a support system." One can be dependent in a healthy way. It is not a sign of weakness to lean on others at times.
- *Don't throw it all away.* Build on what you have. Change is not always the answer, particularly if the problem is internal turmoil. Look before you leap in making job, career, or marital changes. It is usually a good rule of thumb to wait until the emotional turmoil has subsided before making major decisions.
- *Hang in there.* Consistent effort and stick-to-itiveness are important in life. Finish a project, a school degree, or a job and no one can ever take the accomplishment away from you. Much success in life comes from being persistent as others fall off the train along the wayside because they did not have the willpower and the endurance. Don't give up. You never know what will happen next in life. Don't let feelings of depression, helplessness, or fear keep you from moving upstream. Be optimistic.
- *Maintain tradition.* The sharing of tradition is a vital link between generations. Grandparents have a wealth of history to share. Encourage them. The warm feeling of family at holiday time or other occasions are special moments. Share your childhood traditions with your children and start new traditions in your own home.

- *Ask for help.* You don't have to do it all yourself. This includes emotional and physical burdens. For every life-problem there are resources to be tapped for information and suggestions. At every stage of life, mentors are available. Reach out and form these helpful relationships. Parenting is a hard job. Just sharing with other parents can make the process easier. Being a caregiver may drain you emotionally and physically. Know your limits and reach out for aid. Help is available for those of you who suffer from emotional pain and have symptoms of mental illness. Just pick up the phone.
- *Be kind to yourself and to each other.* Life is short. We only pass this way once.

References

Introduction. Midlife: A Perspective

1. Modell, AH: "Object Relations Theory: Psychic Aliveness in the Middle Years," in *The Middle Years: New Psychoanalytic Perspectives*, Oldham, JM, and Liebert, RS, eds. (New Haven: Yale University Press, 1989), pp. 17, 20.
2. Murray, R, and Zentner, J: *Nursing Assessment and Health Promotion through the Life Span* (Englewood Cliffs, NJ: Prentice-Hall, 1975), p. 252.

Chapter 2. The Parent–Child Bond

1. Schuster, CS, and Ashburn, SS: *The Process of Human Development: A Holistic Life-Span Approach*, 2nd ed. (Boston: Little, Brown, 1986), pp. 172, 666–667.
2. McKinney, WT: "Interdisciplinary Animal Research and Its Relevance to Psychiatry," in *Comprehensive Textbook of Psychiatry*, Vol. 1, 5th Ed., Kaplan, HI, and Sadock, BJ, M.D., eds. (Baltimore: Williams & Wilkins, 1989), pp. 327, 336–337.
3. McGee, MG, and Wilson, DW: *Psychology: Science and Application* (New York: West, 1984), pp. 278–279.
4. Freud, S: *The Ego and the Id*, J Strachey, ed. and trans. (New York: Norton, 1960).
5. Erikson, EH: *Childhood and Society*, 2nd ed. (New York: Norton, 1963).
6. Bowlby, J: "The Nature of the Child's Tie to His Mother," *International Journal of Psychoanalysis*, 1958; 39:350–373.
7. Ainsworth, MDS: "Attachment and Dependency: A Comparison,"

in *Attachment and Dependency*, JL Gerwirtz, ed. (Washington, D.C.; Winston, 1972).

8. Goldberg, SR, and Deursch, F: *Life-Span Individual and Family Development* (Monterey, CA: Brooks/Cole, 1977), pp. 298, 303.

9. Klaus, M., et al.: "Maternal Attachment: Importance of the First Post-Partum Days," *New England Journal Medicine*, 1972:286:460.

10. Spitrz, RA, and Wolf, KM: "Anaclitic Depression," in *The Psychoanalytic Study of the Child* (New York: International Universities Press, 1946), Vol. 2, p. 313.

11. Spitz, RA: "Hospitalization: An Inquiry into the Genesis of Psychiatric Conditions in Early Childhood," in *The Psychoanalytic Study of the Child* (New York: International Universities Press, 1945), Vol. 1, pp. 53–74.

12. Benjamin, LT, Jr., Hopkins, JR, and Nation, JR: *Psychology* (New York: Macmillan, 1987), p. 310.

13. Jessner, L, Weigert, E, and Foy, JL: "The Development of Parental Attitudes during Pregnancy," in *Parenthood: Its Psychology and Psychopathology*, EJ Anthony and T Benedek, eds. (Boston: Little, Brown, 1970).

14. Klaus, MH, and Kennell, JH: *Parent–Infant Bonding*, 2nd ed. (St. Louis: Mosby, 1982), p. 3.

15. Bowlby, J: "The Making and Breaking of Affectional Bonds," *British Journal Psychiatry*, 1977:130:201–210.

16. *Psychology Today: An Introduction*, 5th ed. RR Bootzin, EF Loftus, and RB Zajonc (Academic Advisors), (New York: Random House, 1983), pp. 328–329.

17. Cameron, N: *Personality Development and Psychopathology: A Dynamic Approach* (Boston: Houghton Mifflin, 1963), p. 83.

Chapter 3. Adolescence: A Period of Explosive Turbulence

1. Freud, S: *Three Essays on the Theory of Sexuality* (1905) (New York: Basic Books, 1962).

2. Freud, A: *The Ego and the Mechanisms of Defense* (New York: International Universities Press, 1966).

3. Erikson, EH: *Childhood and Society*, 2nd ed. (New York: Norton, 1963).

4. *Psychology Today: An Introduction*, 5th ed. RR Bootzin, EF Loftus, and

RB Zajonc (Academic Advisors) (New York: Random House, 1983), p. 338.

5. Cameron, N: *Personality Development and Psychopathology: A Dynamic Approach* (Boston: Houghton Mifflin, 1963), p. 110.

6. Benjamin, LT, Jr., Hopkins, JR, and Nation, JR: *Psychology* (New York: Macmillan, 1987), p. 355.

7. Erikson, EH: *Identity: Youth and Crisis* (New York: Norton, 1968), p. 105.

8. Zal, HM: "Adolescence—A Period of Explosive Turbulence," *Health,* September, 1967, Vol. 13, No. 1, pp. 6–11. This article by the author serves as the skeletal outline upon which this chapter was based. My thanks to the American Osteopathic Association for permission for its use.

Chapter 4. Troubled Teens

1. Zal, HM: "Teen Suicide," *Osteopathic Medical News,* June, 1987, Vol. 4, No. 6, p. 15.

2. Atala, KD, and Baxter, RF: "Suicidal Adolescents: How to Help Them Before Its Too Late," *Postgraduate Medicine,* October 1989, Vol. 86, No. 5, pp. 223–225, 229–230.

3. Husain, SA: "Current Perspectives on the Role of Psychosocial Factors in Adolescent Suicide," *Psychiatric Annals,* March, 1990, Vol. 20, No. 3, pp. 122–124,127.

4. National Center for Health Statistics: *Monthly Vital Statistics Report,* 1989; 38(5):19,29.

5. *Diagnostic and Statistical Manual of Mental Disorders,* Third Edition-Revised (DSM-III-R) Washington, D.C.: American Psychiatric Association), pp. 218–219.

6. Zal, HM: "Diagnosis and Treatment of Adolescent Depression," *Clinical Advances in the Treatment of Psychiatric Disorders,* January/February 1990, Vol. 4, No. 1, p. 8.

7. Zal, HM: "Recognition and Management of the Suicidal Adolescent," *Family Practice Recertification,* November, 1990, Vol. 12, No. 11, p. 107.

8. Shaffer, D, Garland, A, Gould, M, et al.: "Preventing Teenage Suicide: A Critical Review," *Journal of the American Academy of Child and Adolescent Psychiatry,* 1988; 27(6):675–87.

9. Heacock, DR: "Suicidal Behavior in Black and Hispanic Youth," Psychiatric Annals, March, 1990, Vol. 20, No. 3, pp. 134–136, 139–142.

10. Murphy, GE: "The Physician's Responsibility for Suicide. II. Errors of Omission," Annals of Internal Medicine, 1975; 82:305.

11. Slaby, AE, and McGuire, PL: "Prevention of Child and Adolescent Suicide," Psychiatry Letter (published by Fair Oaks Hospital, Summit, NJ), December, 1986, Vol. 4, Issue 12, pp. 65–72.

12. Garfinkel, B: "Adolescent Suicide," Psychiatry Letter (published by Fair Oaks Hospital, Summit, NJ), December, 1989, Vol. 7, Issue 1, pp. 1–4, 6.

13. Toolan, JM: "Depression in Children and Adolescents," in Adolescence: Psychosocial Perspectives, G Caplan and S Lebovici, eds. (New York: Basic Books, 1969).

14. Zal, HM: "Adolescent Depression: An Overview," Journal of the American Osteopathic Association, December 1971, Vol. 71, pp. 89–95.

15. Chwast, J: "Depressive Reactions as Manifested among Adolescent Delinquents," American Journal of Psychotherapy, July, 1967; 21:575–84.

16. Glaser, K: "Masked Depression in Children and Adolescents," American Journal of Psychotherapy, July, 1967; 21:565–574.

17. Braceland, FJ, and Farnsworth, DL: "Depression in Adolescents and College Students," Maryland Medical Journal, April,1969; 18:67–73.

18. Symonds M: "The Depressions in Childhood and Adolescence," American Journal of Psychoanalysis, 1968; 28:189–95.

19. "AMA Launches National Project on Health Needs of Adolescents," Psychiatric News, January 16, 1987, pp. 1, 6–7.

20. Zal, HM: "Substance Abuse," Osteopathic Medical News, September, 1987, Vol. 4, No. 8, p. 28.

21. Rome, HP: "Personal Reflections: Eating Disorders," Psychiatric Annals, September, 1989, Vol. 19, No. 9, p. 464.

22. Pope, HG, Hudson JI, Yurgelun-Todd D, et al.: "Prevalence of Anorexia Nervosa and Bulimia in Three Student Populations," International Journal Eating Disorders, 1984;3(3):45–51.

23. Hudson, JI, and Pope, HG: "Depression and Eating Disorders," in OG Cameron, ed., Presentations of Depression (New York: Wiley, 1987), pp. 33–66.

24. Crisp, AH: "The Psychopathology of Anorexia Nervosa: Getting the 'Heat' Out of the System," in AJ Stunkard and E Stellar, eds., Eating and Its Disorders (New York: Raven Press, 1984).

25. Ganz, M: "Eating Disorders," *Osteopathic Annals*, November, 1984, Vol. 12, pp. 29–36.

26. Herzog, DB: "An Overview of Eating Disorders," *Advances in Psychiatry: Focus on Eating Disorders* (New York: Park Row Publishers, 1987), p. 7.

27. Zal, HM: "Eating Disorders," *Osteopathic Medical News*, May, 1991, Vol. 8, No. 5, p. 20.

28. Johnson, JM: "Is Schizophrenia Genetically Transmitted?" *Journal of the American Osteopathic Association*, April, 1990, Vol. 90, No. 4, pp. 346–351.

29. "Mental Illnesses Awareness Week Backgrounder," 1990, published by the American Psychiatric Association, Division of Public Affairs, Washington, D.C.

30. Erikson, EH: *Identity: Youth and Crisis* (New York: Norton, 1968), pp. 156–158.

Chapter 5. Young Adulthood:
The Twentysomething Generation

1. Gross, DM, and Scott, S: "Proceeding with Caution," *Time*, July 16, 1990, Vol. 136, No. 3, pp. 56–62.

2. Erikson, EH: "The Problem of Ego Identity," *Journal of the American Psychoanalytic Association*, Vol. 4, 1956.

3. Havighurst, RJ: *Developmental Tasks and Education*, 3rd ed. (New York: McKay, 1972).

4. Levinson, DJ, Darrow, CN, Levison, MH, and McKee, B: *The Seasons of a Man's Life* (New York, Ballantine, 1986), pp. 21, 58–59, 111.

5. Mercer, RT, Nichols, EG, and Doyle, GC: *Transitions in a Woman's Life: Major Life Events in Developmental Context* (New York: Springer, 1989), pp. 11,180.

6. Roberts, P, and Newton, PM: *Levinsonian Studies of Women's Adult Development, Psychology and Aging*, 1987;2:154–163.

7. Stewart, WA: "A Psychosocial Study of the Formation of the Early Adult Life Structure in Women," unpublished doctoral dissertation, Columbia University, New York.

8. Blos, P: *On Adolescence: A Psychoanalytic Interpretation* (New York: Free Press, 1962), pp. 124,157.

9. Gould, RL: "Adulthood," in *Comprehensive Textbook of Psychiatry*, V,

HI Kaplan and BJ Sadock, eds., Vol. 2, 5th ed. (Baltimore: Williams & Wilkins, 1989), p. 2003.

10. Goldberg, SR, and Deutsch, F: *Life-Span Individual and Family Development* (Monterey, CA: Wadsworth, 1977), pp. 258, 314, 320, 322.

11. Erikson, EH: *Identity: Youth and Crisis* (New York: Norton, 1968), pp. 135–136.

12. McGee, MG, and Wilson, DW: *Psychology: Science and Application* (New York: West, 1984), p. 291.

13. Edelhart, M: *Getting from Twenty to Thirty: Surviving Your First Decade in the Real World* (New York: Evans, 1983), pp. 103,105,154.

14. Lederer, WJ, and Jackson, DD: *The Mirages of Marriage* (New York: Norton, 1968).

15. Sheehy, G: *Passages: Predictable Crises of Adult Life* (New York: Dutton, 1976), pp. 97–159,163–164.

16. Zal, HM: "Adjusting to Parenthood," *Osteopathic Medical News*, November/December 1987, Vol. 4, No. 10, p. 50.

Chapter 6. Anxiety and Other Emotional Roadblocks in Young Adulthood

1. Mercer RT, Nichols, EG, and Doyle, GC: *Transitions in a Woman's Life: Major Life Events in Developmental Context* (New York: Springer, 1989), p. 3.

2. McGlynn, TJ, and Metcalf, HL, eds.: *Diagnosis and Treatment of Anxiety Disorders: A Physician's Handbook*, 1989 (Washington, D.C.: American Psychiatric Press), pp. 53–57.

3. Zal, HM: *Panic Disorder: The Great Pretender* (New York: Plenum/ Insight, 1990), pp. 61,112.

4. Goodwin, DW: *Anxiety* (New York: Oxford University Press, 1986), p. 114.

5. Thyer, BA, Parrish, RT, Curtis, GC, et al.: "Ages of Onset of DSM-III Anxiety Disorders," *Comprehensive Psychiatry*, 1985, 26:113–122.

6. Erikson, EH: *Identity: Youth and Crisis* (New York: Norton, 1968), p. 136.

7. Perry, JC, and Vaillant, GE: "Personality Disorders," in *Comprehensive Textbook of Psychiatry/V*, HI Kaplan and BJ Sadock, eds, Vol. 2, 5th ed. (Baltimore: Williams & Wilkins, 1989), pp. 1355–1357.

8. Roberts, P, and Newton, PM: "Levinsonian Studies of Women's Adult Development," *Psychology and Aging*, 1987; 2:154–163.

9. Levinson, DJ, Darrow, CN, Klein, EB, et al.: *The Seasons of Man's Life* (New York: Knopf, 1985), pp. 58–59.
10. Sheehy, G: *Passages: Predictable Crises of Adult Life* (New York: Dutton, 1976), pp. 163–164.
11. Rosenmayr, L, and Kockeis, E: "Propositions for a Sociological Theory of Aging and the Family," *International Social Science Journal*, 1963;15:410–426.
12. Goldberg, SR, and Deutsch, F: *Life Span Individual and Family Development* (Monterey, CA: Wadsworth, 1977), p. 314.

Chapter 7. The Challenge of Middle Age

1. *Psychology Today: An Introduction*, 5th ed. RR Bootzin, EF Loftus, and RB Zajonc (Academic Advisors) (New York: Random House, 1983), pp. 338, 500.
2. Wloszczyna, S: "Comic Born of the Trials of Parenting: Middle-Aged Menace," *USA Today*, October 19, 1990, pp. 1D–2D.
3. Sifford, D: "Midlife Crisis: 'The Nagging Pain of Unfulfilled Dreams,' " *Philadelphia Inquirer*, October 17, 1983, p. 4-F.
4. Zal, HM: "The Climacterium and Midlife Crisis," *Osteopathic Annals*, February, 1984, Vol. 12, No. 2, pp. 67–73.
5. Cooke, CW, and Dworkin, S: *The Ms. Guide to a Woman's Health* (New York: Berkeley, 1981), pp. 301–318.
6. Sharma, VK, and Saxena, MS: "Climacteric Symptoms: A Study in the Indian Context," *Maturitas*, 1981; 3:11–20.
7. Townsend, JM, and Carbone, CL: "Menopausal Syndrome: Illness or Social Role—A Transcultural Analysis," *Cultural Medicine and Psychiatry*, 1980; 4:229–248.
8. Greenblatt, RB: "The Other Symptoms of Menopause," *Diagnosis*, 1982; 4:99–103.
9. Luckmann, J, and Sorenson, KC: *Medical Surgical Nursing: A Psychophysiologic Approach* (Philadelphia: Saunders, 1974), pp. 1,407–408.
10. Klein HR: "Obstetrical and Gynecological Disorders," in AM Freedman and HI Kaplan, eds., *Comprehensive Textbook of Psychiatry* (Baltimore: Williams & Wilkins, 1967), pp. 76–84.
11. Schwartz, LH, and Schwartz, JL: *The Psychodynamics of Patient Care* (Englewood Cliffs, NJ: Prentice-Hall, 1972), pp. 305–310.
12. Clegborn, RA, and McClure, DJ: "Endocrines," in A Freedman and

HI Kaplan, eds., *Comprehensive Textbook of Psychiatry* (Baltimore: Williams & Wilkins, 1967), pp. 85–93.

13. Polit, DF, and LaRocco, SA: "Social and Psychological Correlates of Menopausal Symptoms," *Psychosomatic Medicine,* 1980; 42:335–45.

14. Coulam CB: "Age, Estrogens, and the Psyche," *Clinical Obstetrics and Gynecology,* 1981;24:219–29.

15. Lurie, HJ: *Clinical Psychiatry for the Primary Physician* (Nutley, NJ: Hoffmann-La Roche, Inc., 1978), pp. 30–31,51–53.

16. McGee, MG, and Wilson, DW: *Psychology: Science and Application* (New York: West, 1984), p. 291.

17. Wiener, MF: "Theories of Personality and Psychopathology: Other Psychodynamic Schools," in HI Kaplan and BJ Sadock, eds., *Comprehensive Textbook of Psychiatry,* Vol. 1, 5th ed. (Baltimore: Williams & Wilkins, 1989), p. 415.

18. Schuster, CS, and Ashburn, SS: *The Process of Human Development: A Holistic Life-Span Approach,* 2nd ed. (Boston: Little, Brown, 1986), p. 758.

19. Erikson, EH: *Childhood and Society,* 2nd ed. (New York: Norton, 1963).

20. Goldberg, SR, and Deutsch, F: *Life-Span Individual and Family Development* (Monterey, CA: Wadsworth, 1977), p. 257.

21. Benjamin, LT, Jr., Hopkins, JR, and Nation, JR: *Psychology* (New York: Macmillan, 1987), p. 355.

22. Erikson, EH: *Identity: Youth and Crisis* (New York: Norton, 1968), p. 105.

23. Levinson, DJ, Darrow, CN, Klein, EB, et al.: *Seasons of a Man's Life* (New York: Knopf, 1985).

24. Duke, MP, and Nowicki, S, Jr.: "Theories of Personality and Psychopathology: Schools Derived from Psychology and Philosophy," in HI Kaplan and BJ Sadock, eds., *Comprehensive Textbook of Psychiatry,* Volume 1, 5th ed. (Baltimore: Williams & Wilkins, 1989), pp. 443–444.

Chapter 8. Crisis Points in Middle Age

1. Wykert, J: "Male Mid-Life Crisis Subject of Intense Debate among Researchers," *Psychiatric News,* September 16, 1983, pp. 22, 35.

2. Wingerd, WN, and Gruber, GR: "Parents Can Have Problems Too," in *Understanding and Enjoying Adolescence* (New York: Longman, 1988), pp. 37, 41.

3. Zal, HM: "Four Stages of Life, Part I," *Osteopathic Medical News,* July/August, 1988, Vol. V, No. 7, p. 28.

4. Bornstein, R: "Cognitive and Psychosocial Development in Middlescence," in CS Schuster and SS Ashburn, eds., *The Process of Human Development: A Holistic Life-Span Approach,* 2nd ed. (Boston: Little, Brown, 1986), p. 768.

5. Deutscher, I: "The Quality of Postparental Life: Definitions of the Situation," *Journal of Marriage and the Family,* 1964; 26:52–59.

6. Zal, HM: *Panic Disorder: The Great Pretender* (New York: Plenum/ Insight, 1990), pp. 165–166.

7. Berne, E: *Games People Play* (New York: Grove Press, 1964).

8. Ben-Gal Kramer, D: "Big Boys Don't Cry: And That's a Big Part of the Problem," *Delaware Valley Magazine,* December, 1990, Vol. 9, No. 8, p. 45.

9. Sifford, D: "Midlife Crisis: The 'Popular Notion' and the Reality," *The Philadelphia Inquirer,* February 13, 1990, p. 10-E.

10. Sifford, D: "The Fading Dreams of Middle-Aged Men," *The Philadelphia Inquirer,* February 19, 1989, pp. 1-K, 9-K.

Chapter 9. The Middle-Aged Mind and Body

1. Horowitz, MH: "The Developmental and Structural Viewpoints: On the Fate of Unconscious Fantasies of Middle Life," in *The Middle Years: New Psychoanalytic Perspectives,* JM Oldham and RS Liebert, eds. (New Haven: Yale University Press, 1989), pp. 7–16.

2. Liebert, RS, and Oldham, JM, eds.: *The Middle Years: New Psychoanalytic Perspectives* (New Haven: Yale University Press, 1989), p. 2.

3. Zal, M: "The Female Alcoholic: Different Problems but the Same Addiction," *Main Line Times Sunday,* September 21, 1986, p. 26.

4. Zal, M: "The Climacterium and Midlife Crisis," *Osteopathic Annals,* February, 1984, Vol. 12, pp. 67–73.

5. Connell, EB (moderator): "Roundtable: Current Understanding of Menstruation and Menopause," *Medical Aspects of Human Sexuality,* 1982;16:440–44.

6. Meyers, H: "The Impact of Teenaged Children on Parents," in *The Middle Years: New Psychoanalytic Perspectives,* JM Oldham and RS Liebert, eds. (New Haven: Yale University Press, 1989), p. 85.

7. "High Blood Pressure," in *Compendium of Patient Information,* ES Geffner (Editor-in-Chief) (New York: McGraw-Hill, 1988).

8. "Learning to Live with Hypertension" (Boston: Medicine in the Public Interest, Inc., 1985), pp. 3–35.

9. Conaway, DC, and Myers, AR: "Rheumatic Disease," in *Medicine*, AR Myers, ed. (New York: Wiley, 1986), pp. 387–390.

10. "Menopause," in *Compendium of Patient Information*, ES Geffner (Editor-in-Chief), (New York: McGraw-Hill, 1988).

11. Cooke, CW, and Dworkin, S: *The Ms. Guide to a Woman's Health* (New York: Berkeley, 1981), pp. 301–318.

12. *Guide to Clinical Preventive Services*, Report of the U.S. Preventive Services Task Force, M Fisher, ed. (Baltimore: Williams & Wilkins, 1989), pp. lii–liii.

13. Zal, HM: "Four Stages of Life, Part I," *Osteopathic Medical News*, July/August, 1988, Vol. V, No. 7, p. 28.

Chapter 10. Middle-Aged Children and Their Aging Parents

1. Blos, P: *On Adolescence: A Psychoanalytic Interpretation* (New York: Free Press, 1962).

2. Oldham, JM: "The Third Individuation," in *The Middle Years: New Psychoanalytic Perspectives*, JM Oldham and RS Liebert, eds. (New Haven: Yale University Press, 1989), pp. 89–104.

3. Zal, HM: *Panic Disorder: The Great Pretender* (New York: Plenum Press/Insight, 1990), pp. 111–112.

4. Viorst, J: "Life Changes—How to Be a Good Parent to Your Parents," *Redbook*, September, 1988, p. 237.

5. Sifford, D: "Midlife Crisis: The 'Popular Notion' and the Reality," *The Philadelphia Inquirer*, February 13, 1990, p. 10-E.

6. Deutsch, F, Popp, CA, Goldberg, SR: "Family Climate: Parent/Child Interactions Over the Life Span," in SR Goldberg and F. Deutsch, eds., *Life-Span: Individual and Family Development* (Monterey, CA: Wadsworth Company, Inc.), p. 322.

7. "The Matter of Midlife Crisis" in the Psychology section of *Health and Fitness*, MaryPat McWilliams, Managing Editor, General Learning Corporation, Highland Park, IL, December 1985/January 1986, pp. 24–25.

8. Jacques, E: "Death and the Mid-Life Crisis," *International Journal of Psychoanalysis*, 1965;46:502–514.

9. Modell, AH: "Object Relations Theory: Psychic Aliveness in the Mid-

dle Years," in JM Oldham and RS Liebert, eds., *The Middle Years: New Psychoanalytic Perspectives* (New Haven: Yale University Press, 1989), p. 21.

10. Gonda, TA: "Death, Dying, and Bereavement," in HI Kaplan and BJ Sadock, eds., *Comprehensive Textbook of Psychiatry/V*, Vol. 2, 5th ed. (Baltimore: Williams & Wilkins, 1989), pp. 1340–1341.

11. Kübler-Ross, E: *On Death and Dying* (New York: Macmillan, 1969).

Chapter 11. The Golden Years

1. Butler, RN: "Psychosocial Aspects of Aging," in HI Kaplan and BJ Sadock, *Comprehensive Textbook of Psychiatry/V*, Vol. 2, 5th ed. (Baltimore: Williams & Wilkins, 1989), pp. 2014–2019.

2. McGee, MG, and Wilson, DW: *Psychology: Science and Application* (New York: West, 1984), pp. 292–293.

3. Erickson, EH: *Childhood and Society,* 2nd ed. (New York: Norton, 1963).

4. Collins, M: *Communication in Health Care* (St. Louis: Mosby, 1977), pp. 105–106.

5. Gould, RL: "Adulthood," in *Comprehensive Textbook of Psychiatry/V,* HI Kaplan and BJ Sadock, eds., Vol. 2, 5th ed. (Baltimore: Williams & Wilkins, 1989), pp. 2006–2007.

6. Zal, HM: "Understanding the Elderly," *Osteopathic Medical News,* March, 1986, Vol. 3, No. 3, p. 47.

7. Sifford, D: "Mining the Pleasures of the 'Golden Years,' " *The Philadelphia Inquirer,* June 28, 1990, p. 5-E.

8. Goldberg, SR, and Deutsch, F: *Life-Span Individual and Family Development* (Monterey, CA: Brooks/Cole, 1977), pp. 318–319.

9. Schuster, CS, and Ashburn, SS: *The Process of Human Development: A Holistic Life-Span Approach,* 2nd ed. (Boston: Little, Brown, 1986), pp. 769–771.

10. Pollock, GH: "Old Age: The Last Development Challenge," in *Aspects of Aging,* Unit I, Psychological Issues, Report No. 2 (Philadelphia: SmithKline Beckman Corp., 1984).

11. Mercer, RT, Nichols, EG, and Doyle, GC: *Transitions in a Woman's Life: Major Life Events in Developmental Context* (New York: Springer, 1989), pp. 167–178.

12. Lopata, HZ: *Widowhood in an American City* (Cambridge, MA: Schenkman, 1973).

13. My thanks to TLA-Central, Wynnewood, Pennsylvania, and the Rev.

John E. Fitzgerald, St. Margaret's Parish, Narberth, Pennsylvania, for permission to use this material.

14. Walters, J: "The Wall of Silence: Sexuality and the Aged," in *Advice for Adults with Aging Parents*, August/September, 1987, Vol 2, No. 4, pp. 5–7. Helpful Publications, Inc., Glenside, Pennsylvania.

15. Fletcher, DJ: "Counseling Elderly Patients about Sex," *Geriatric Consultant*, September/October, 1982, Vol. 1, No. 2, pp. 20–24.

16. Strauss, D: "Aging and Old Age" in *Understanding Human Behavior in Health and Illness*, RC Simons and H Pardes, eds. (Baltimore: Williams & Wilkins, 1977), pp. 373–374.

Chapter 12. The Last Mile

1. Zal, HM: "Understanding the Elderly," *Osteopathic Medical News*, March, 1986, Vol. 3, No. 3, pp. 1,47–49.

2. US Census Bureau, Washington, D.C.

3. Kaufman, M: "Becoming 'Old, Old,'" *The Philadelphia Inquirer*, p. 10-A.

4. *Webster's New World Dictionary of the American Language*, College Ed. (New York: World, 1957), p. 389.

5. Zal, HM: "Geriatric Psychiatry—Growing Older in the 80's," *Osteopathic Annals*, January, 1983, Vol. 11, No. 1, pp. 50–51.

6. Billing, N: *To Be Old and Sad: Understanding Depression in the Elderly* (Lexington, MA: Lexington Books Heath, 1987), p. 69.

7. "Mental Health of the Elderly," A "Let's Talk Facts About" pamphlet (Washington, D.C.: American Psychiatric Association, 1988), p. 2.

8. Zal, HM: "Depression in the Elderly Patient," in *Difficult Medical Management*, RB Taylor, ed. (Philadelphia: Saunders, 1991), pp. 187–194.

9. Thomas, P: "Primary Care: Depressed Elderly's Best Hope," *Medical World News*, July 13, 1987, pp. 39–54.

10. *Diagnostic and Statistical Manual of Mental Disorders* Third Edition-Revised (DSM-III-R) (Washington, D.C.: American Psychiatric Association, 1987).

11. Jarvik, LF: "Depression: A Review of Drug Therapy for Elderly Patients," *Consultant*, 1982; 22:141–146.

12. Thienhaus, OJ: "Depression in the Elderly: Phenomenology and Pharmacotherapy, *Geriatric Medicine Today*, 1989;8:34–45.

13. Butler, RH: "Psychological Aspects of Aging," *Comprehensive Text-

book of Psychiatry/V, Vol. 2, 5th ed., HI Kaplan and BJ Sadock, eds. (Baltimore: Williams & Wilkins, 1989), pp. 2014–2019.

14. "When You Need a Nursing Home," *Age Page*, National Institute on Aging, U.S. Department of Health and Human Services, November, 1986.

15. Michels, KA: "Meeting the Challenges of Care in the Nursing Home," *Family Practice Recertification*, February, 1991, Vol. 13, No. 2, pp. 33–48.

16. Macee NL, and Rabins, PV: *The 36-Hour Day: A Family Guide to Caring for Persons with Alzheimer's Disease, Related Dementing Illnesses, and Memory Loss in Later Life* (Baltimore: Johns Hopkins University Press, 1981), p. 193.

17. Baker, FM, Perr, IN, and Yesavage, JA: *An Overview of Legal Issues in Geriatric Psychiatry*, Report of the American Psychiatric Association Task Force on Forensic Issues in Geriatric Psychiatry, (Washington, D.C.: American Psychiatric Association, 1986). p. 1.

18. Viorst, J: "Life Changes—How to Be a Good Parent to Your Parents," *Redbook*, September, 1988, pp. 158–159, 234, 237.

19. Holtzman, P: "When Child and Parent Switch Roles," *The Philadelphia Inquirer*, January 27, 1986, p. 2–3-M.

20. Weinberg, J: "What Do I Say to My Mother When I Have Nothing to Say?", *Geriatrics*, November 1974, pp. 155–159.

21. Thunberg, U: "Death and the Dying Adult," in *Understanding Human Behavior in Health and Illness*, R Simons and H. Pardes, eds. (Baltimore: Williams & Wilkins, 1977), p. 392.

Chapter 13. Middle-Aged Wisdom

1. Kushner, HS: *When All You've Ever Wanted Isn't Enough* (New York: Summit Books, 1986), pp. 141,190.

2. Frosch, WA: "Toward a Definition of Psychiatry," *Psychiatric News*, April 19, 1991, Vol. 26, No. 8, p. 38.

3. Goodman, A: "Organic Unity Theory: The Mind-Body Problem Revisited," *American Journal of Psychiatry*, May, 1991, 148:5:553–563.

4. Gelman, D, and Hager, M: "Body and Soul." *Newsweek*, November 7, 1988, pp. 88–97.

5. Reiman, EM, Raichle, ME, Robbins, E, et al.: "The Application of Positron Emission Tomography to the Study of Panic Disorder," *American Journal of Psychiatry*, 1986;143:469–471.

6. Zal, HM: *Panic Disorder: The Great Pretender* (New York: Plenum/ Insight, 1990), p. 114.
7. Zal, HM: "Substance Abuse," *Osteopathic Medical News*, September, 1987, Vol. 4, No. 8, p. 28.
8. Dryden, J: "Alexander's Feast" (1697), line 58.

Index

Abuse, by parents, 161–162
Acceptance, need for, 221
Addiction, as stress symptom, 56–57
Adolescence. *See also* Parent–child relationship; Young adulthood
behavioral inconsistencies in, 42–44
career choices in, 37
changes during, 31–32
depression in, 48, 50, 53, 54–56
developmental tasks, 33–39
eating disorders in, 58–61
experimentation needs, 65–66
generation gap and, 39–40
group membership in, 38
identity search in, 36–38
mental health treatment, 63–66
parental understanding of, 40–46
physical development during, 33–34
psychodynamic system of, 43
psychological changes in, 34
reassurance needs in, 33–34
rebellion during, 36, 55

Adolescence (*cont.*)
role models, 38–39
schizophrenia in, 61–63
separation from parents, 34–36
substance abuse in, 56–58
turmoil during, 42–44
vignettes, 32–33, 36
Adolescent suicide. *See* Suicide
Adulthood. *See* Late adulthood; Young adulthood
Affairs, extramarital, 122–124
Aging parents. *See also* Elderly
midlife children and, 155–170
Ainsworth, Mary, 19, 20
Alanon, 58
Ala-Teen, 58
Alcoholics Anonymous (AA), 58
Alcoholism, in adolescents, 56
Alzheimer, Alois, 192
Alzheimer's disease, 192
American Association of Retired Persons, 178
Anaclitic depression, *See* Depression
Anatomy of an Illness (Cousins), 222

241

Anger, in relationships, 125–126
Anorexia nervosa, 60
Anxiety
  health worries and, 142–144
  in midlife, 135–136
  stress related, 130–134
Anxiety disorders
  vignettes, 86, 87–88, 89, 91
  in young adulthood, 85–91
Aristotle, 181
Arthritis, 146–147
Attachment. *See also* Separation
    defined, 15–16
  developmental stages and,
    18–19, 20
  maternal deprivation and,
    21–22
  theories of, 17–20

Babies. *See* Infants
Baby boomers, 100
Bach, Johann S., 181
Back pain, 146
Beethoven, van, Ludwig, 181
Berne, Eric, 131
Bipolar disorders. *See* Manic-
    depressive illness
Blacks, suicide rate, 49–50
Body–mind relationship, 218
Bonding. *See also* Parent–child
    bonding
  animal models, 16
  defined, 15–16
  significant others and, 22–23
Borderline personality disorder.
    See Personality disorders
Bowlby, John, 15, 19, 20
Bradshaw, John, 112, 158
Brain syndromes, reversible, 192

Browning, Robert, 194
Bulimia nervosa, 61

Career choices
  adolescents, 37
  midlife, 118–120, 126–127
  parental reactions to, 37, 74
  young adults, 73–74
Caregivers
  avoiding burnout, 205–209
  role for children of elderly,
    203–209
Chagall, Marc, 181
Child development. *See also* De-
    velopmental tasks
  early childhood, 24–26
  infancy, 23–24
  latency age children, 26
  oedipal conflicts and, 25–26
  theories of, 17–20
Child within perspective, 112, 158
Children. *See also* Infants; Parent–
    child bonding; Parent–child
    relationship
  care of elderly parents, 203–209
  love needs, 79
  view of parents, 160–163
Chinese, attitudes toward eld-
    erly, 190
Cholesterol, levels, 145–146
Collective unconscious, 107
College students
  depression among, 55–56
  parents' views of, 69–71
  substance abuse by, 57
Commitment, involuntary, 64–65
Communication
  parent–child relationship and,
    34, 41–42, 43–44, 45

Communication (*cont.*)
    as stress reducer, 131–132
Community resources, for eld-
    erly, 176
Compulsive disorder. *See* Obses-
    sive-compulsive disorder
Conservatorships, 202–203
Contact comfort, 16, 23
Coping guidelines. *See* Guidelines
Couples therapy
    divorce prevention, 124–128
    hidden agendas in, 121–122
    past issues and, 126
    willingness to attend, 127
Cousins, Norman, 222
Creativity, in late life, 176,
    180–182
Criticism, accepting, 221
Culture, suicide and, 49–50

Death
    of elderly, 209–210
    midlife perspective, 166–167
    of parent, 167–169, 209–210
    rituals of, 210
    of spouse, 182–185
Degenerative joint disease (DJD).
    See Osteoarthritis
Delinquency, as depression symp-
    tom, 55
Delusional disorder, 138–139
Dementia
    in elderly, 190–194, 196
    vignette, 193–194
Dementia praecox. *See* Schizo-
    phrenia
Depression. *See also* Manic-
    depressive illness
    anaclitic, 21

Depression (*cont.*)
    anxiety disorders and, 87
    dementia and, 196
    eating disorders and, 60
    in elderly, 194–196
    job related, 118
    masked, 54–56, 195
    in midlife, 136–139
    stress and, 130
    substance abuse and, 56
    suicide and, 48, 50, 53, 55
    symptoms, 54–56, 137–139
Descartes, Rene, 218
Developmental tasks. *See also* At-
    tachment; Child develop-
    ment; Parent–child bonding
    adolescents, 33–39
    late adulthood, 173–174
    middle age, 101–102, 105–110
    young adulthood, 68–69, 73–79
Diabetes, adult onset, 148
*Diagnostic and Statistical Manual
    of Mental Disorders* (DSM-
    III-R), 195
Divorce
    in midlife, 121
    prevention of, 124–128
Do not resuscitate decisions
    (DNR), 203
Dryden, John, 222
Dysthymia. *See* Depression

Eating disorders
    adolescents, 58–61
    vignette, 58–60
Edison, Thomas, 181
Elderhostel, 178
Elderly. *See also* Aging parents;
    Late adulthood

Elderly (*cont.*)
 attitudes toward, 189–190
 caregiver role of children,
  203–209
 death of, 209–210
 dementia in, 190–193, 196
 depression in, 194–196
 guardianship for, 202–203
 hypochondriacal complaints,
  191
 legal concerns, 201–203
 living arrangements, 196–199
 placement in nursing homes,
  199–201
 population figures, 190
 support systems for, 206–207
 understanding of, 190–191
 vignette, 189
Emerson, Ralph W., 40, 44, 113
Emotional pressures, of young
  adulthood, 85–95
Empty bucket syndrome. *See* Personality disorders
Empty nest syndrome, 128–130
Erikson, Erik
 on adolescence, 65, 67–68
 developmental theories, 18–19,
  20, 37, 75
 on late adulthood, 173, 182
 on midlife, 107–108, 110
Exams, medical, 148–151
Exercise, midlife needs, 152

Family disruption, suicide and,
  48–49
Family pressure, career choice
  and, 118–120

Fathers. *See also* Parent–child
  bonding; Parent–child rela-
  tionship
 caretaker role, 22–23
Firestone, Harvey, 181
Ford, Henry, 181
Freud, Anna, 35, 37
Freud, Sigmund, 17, 20, 34, 37,
  93, 106, 181
Friendship, elements of, 40

Gender role, development of, 25
Generalized anxiety disorder
  (GAD). *See* Anxiety disorders
Generation gap, 39–40
Generations, similarity of wants
  and needs, 219–222
Gordon, Ruth, 181
Graham, Martha, 181
Grandparenthood, 179–180
Grieving process, 168–169,
  183–185
Guardianship, for elderly,
  202–203
Guidelines
 for adolescent mental health
  needs, 63–66
 for adolescent substance abus-
  ers, 57–58
 for bonding success, 20–21
 for care of elderly, 207–209
 for midlife success, 110–113,
  151–153, 223–226
 for parent–child relationship,
  44–46, 82–83, 169–170
 for stress reduction, 133–134
 for suicide prevention, 51–54

Harlow, Harry, 16, 19, 20, 22

Harlow, Margaret, 16
Health, in midlife, 142–154
Health exams, 148–151
Hispanics, suicide rate, 49–50
Hobbes, Thomas, 218
Hobbies, for elderly, 176
Home, leaving, 69–71, 72–73, 81
Home health care, 198
Honesty, need for, 222
Hope, need for, 222
Hopelessness, suicide and, 51
Hospitalism, 21
Housing, for elderly, 196–199
Hypercholesterolemia, described, 145–146
Hypertension, described, 145

Identity crisis, in adolescence, 36–38
Imprinting, defined, 16
Incontinence, stress, 148
India, attitudes toward elderly, 190
Individualization, 107, 109
Infants
    institutionalized, 21
    maternal deprivation of, 21–22
    parent–child bonding and, 20–21, 23–24
Integrity, in late life, 182
Interventions. *See* Therapy
Intimacy
    achievement of, 75
    need for, 221–222
    personality disorders and, 94
Involuntary commitment, 64–65

Jaques, Elliott, 167
Jefferson, Thomas, 222

Jolly Roger Syndrome, 115–117.
    See also Midlife crisis
Jung, Carl, 107, 110
Ketcham, Hank, 100
Kushner, Rabbi Harold, 212

Laboratory tests, 150–151
Late adulthood. *See also* Elderly
    creativity in, 176, 180–182
    developmental tasks of, 173–174
    family involvement, 177–178
    needs of, 187–188
    sexual activity in, 185–187
    travel in, 178
    vignette, 174–175
    volunteerism in, 177
    work in, 177
Leibnitz, von, Gottfried, 218
Levinson, Daniel J., 73, 108–109
"Listen" (anonymous), 41–42
Living arrangements
    for elderly, 196–199
    vignette, 196
Living wills, 202
Longfellow, Henry Wadsworth, 180–181
Lorenz, Konrad, 16, 20
Losses, suicide and, 48
Love
    bonding and, 20
    Freud on, 93
    mature, 22, 75–76, 220–221
    need for, 79, 221
    roadblocks to, 125–126
    in young adults, 74–76
Love object relationships. *See* Object relationships

Male climacteric, 104–105
Manic-depressive illness, 91–93
Marital counseling. *See* Couples
      therapy
Marriage
   age factors, 76
   midlife crisis and, 120–128
   reasons for, 76
   suggestions for, 76–77
   in young adulthood, 76–77
Masked depression. *See* Depres-
      sion
Maslow, Abraham, 109–110
Medical exams, 148–151
Melancholic depression. *See* De-
      pression
Men. *See also* Fathers; Male cli-
      macteric
   sexual issues, 141–142
Menopause, 102–104
   attitudes toward, 103
   cultural aspects, 102
   described, 147–148
   sexual activity and, 141–142
   symptoms, 103–104
Mental health groups, 132–133
Mental health therapy. *See* Ther-
      apy
Mental illness, attitudes toward,
      217–218
"Mental Notes with Dr. Michael
      Zal," 183
Michaelangelo Buonarroti, 181
Middle age. *See also* Male climac-
      teric; Menopause; Midlife
      crisis
   aging parents in, 155–170
   anxieties of, 135–136
   depression in, 136–139

Middle age (*cont.*)
   developmental tasks, 101–102,
      105–110
   dilemmas of, 100–102
   failed expectations of, 213–214
   generativity vs. stagnation in,
      107–108
   health exams, 148–151
   health issues, 142–154
   mortality issues, 166–167
   personal growth in, 106–113
   personality integration in,
      110–111
   perspectives on, 211–213
   physical disorders of, 144–148
   population numbers, 100
   productiveness goals, 107–108
   relationships in, 109, 112,
      120–128
   relaxation in, 111
   sexual issues, 140–142
   stagnation in, 108
   standing alone in, 155–156
   as state of mind, 101
   stress in, 130–134
   substance abuse in, 139–140
   success guidelines, 110–113,
      151–153, 223–226
   theories of, 105–110
   usefulness concerns, 106
   vignettes, 7–13, 99–100
   work in, 112
Midlife crisis
   aging parents and, 155, 166
   defined, 101
   destructive choices, 116–117
   marriage issues, 120–128
   men, 105, 120–128
   relationship issues, 120–128

Midlife crisis (*cont.*)
  vignettes, 115–116, 119–120, 123–124
  women, 108, 120–128
  work stress and, 117–120
Mind–body relationship, 218
Mirages of Marriage, The (Jackson and Lederer), 76
"Morituri Salutamus" (Longfellow), 180–181
Mortality, midlife perspective, 166–167
Mothers. *See also* Parent–child bonding; Parent–child relationship
  deprivation of infants, 21–22
  status of, 74

Narcotics Anonymous (NA), 58
National Institute on Alcohol Abuse and Alcoholism (NIAAA), 56
National Support Center for Families of the Aging, 198
Necessary Losses (Viorst), 157
Need theory, 16
Needs
  levels of, 110
  universal, 219–222
  verbalizing of, 125
Nursing homes
  benefits of, 200
  choosing, 199–201
  numbers in, 197
  placement in, 199–201
  problems with, 201
  sexual activity in, 187
Nutrition, midlife needs, 151–152

Obesity, menopause symptoms and, 104
Object relationships, 17, 21–22, 23
Obsessive-compulsive disorder (OCD), 89–90
Occupational choices. *See* Career choices
Oedipal conflicts, child development and, 25–26
Old age. *See* Elderly
Ormandy, Eugene, 181
Osteoarthritis, described, 146–147

Pain, need to be free of, 222
Panic disorder, 87–89, 218
Parent–child bonding, 15–27
  with aged parents, 155–170
  clinical vignette, 17–18
  development and, 20
  in early childhood, 24–26
  fathers and, 22–23
  guidelines, 20–21
  in infancy, 23–24
  in latency age children, 26
  maternal deprivation and, 21–22
  personality development and, 24
  in young adulthood, 80–83, 95
Parent–child relationship
  acceptance of parent, 79–80, 160–163, 165
  achieving a new relationship, 158–160, 164–165
  in adolescence, 32, 33–34, 40–46
  career choice and, 37, 74
  college students, 69–71

Parent–child relationship (*cont.*)
  communication and, 34, 41–42,
    43–44, 45
  empty nest syndrome, 128–130
  favoritism by parent, 162–163
  grandparenthood, 179–180
  leaving home and, 69–71,
    72–73
  resolving old issues, 158–160,
    164–165
  with retired parents, 175–179
  role reversal, 156–157
  separation from parents,
    34–36, 69–71, 72–73, 129
  success guidelines, 169–170
  suicide prevention and, 51–54
  vignettes, 159–160, 163–164
  in young adulthood, 69–71,
    79–83
Parenthood
  adjusting to, 77–79
  vignette, 77–78
  in young adulthood, 76–77
Parents. *See also* Aging parents;
    Parent–child bonding; Par-
    ent–child relationship
  abusive behavior by, 161–162
  adolescent sexuality and, 142
  adolescent substance abuse
    and, 57–58
  appreciation of, 79–80
  care of elderly, 203–209
  death of, 166, 167–169, 209–210
  need to grow, 41–42
  toxic, 165
Passages (Sheehy), 76
Peer groups, 38
Personality
  development of, 24, 25

Personality (*cont.*)
  integration of, 110–111
Personality disorders, 17, 21–22,
    23, 93–94
Phobias, 90–91
Physical examinations, 150
Picasso, Pablo, 181
Postadolescence. *See* Young adult-
    hood
Power of attorney, 202
Pseudodementia, 196
Psychiatrist, defined, 215
Psychosis. *See also* Manic-
    depressive illness; Schizo-
    phrenia
  development of, 17
  suicide and, 49
Psychosocial development. *See*
    Child development
Psychotherapy. *See* Therapy
Psychotic depressive reaction.
    See Depression

Race, suicide and, 49–50
Reactive depression. *See*
    Depression
Rebelliousness, as depression
    symptom, 55
Recovery, Inc., 133
Recreation, in middle age, 111
Relationships. *See also* Couples
    therapy
  in middle age, 109, 112
  midlife crisis and, 120–128
  suggestions for, 76–77
Relaxation, in middle age, 111
Rembrandt, 181
Residential care facilities, 197
Respect, need for, 222

Retirement
   approaches to, 111, 175–179
   vignette, 174–175
Retirement homes, 197
Role models
   for adolescents, 38–39
   parents as, 67

Sandwich generation. *See* Middle
   age
Schizophrenia
   adolescents, 61–63
   symptoms, 62
   vignette, 61
Seasons of a Man's Life, The
   (Levinson), 73, 108–109
Self-concept, in adolescence, 35
Self-actualization, 110
Self-realization, 107
Self-transcendence, 110
Senility, 190–191
Senior citizen groups, 176
Separation. *See also* Attachment
   adolescents from parents, 34–36
   anxiety, 24
   young adults from parents,
      69–71, 72–73, 129
Sex differences, in development,
   73
Sex role, development of, 25
Sexual issues
   in late adulthood, 185–187
   in middle age, 104–105,
      140–142
   in nursing homes, 187
Sheehy, Gail, 76
Sibling rivalry, 162–163
Sifford, Darrell, 101

Significant others, bonding and,
   22–23
Social phobias, 90–91
Socialization, 25
Spitz, Rene, 21
Spouse, death of, 182–185
Stevenson, Adlai, 211
Stress
   addiction as symptom, 56–57
   in midlife, 130–134
   physical illness and, 130
   reduction techniques, 130–134
   substance abuse and, 56–57,
      140
   work related, 117–120
Substance abuse
   in adolescents, 56–58
   in midlife, 139–140
   parental guidance, 57–58
   personality disorders and, 94
   vignette, 139–140
Suicide
   of adolescents, 47–48, 49–50
   cluster suicide, 50
   cultural factors, 49–50
   of elderly, 194
   family history of, 49
   prevention, 51–54
   racial factors, 49–50
   risk factors, 48–50
   vignette, 47
   warning signs, 50–51
Support systems, for elderly,
   206–207
Systems review, in health exams,
   149–150

Teenagers. *See* Adolescence
Terminally ill, 210

Therapy. *See also* Couples therapy
  for adolescents, 63–66
  benefits of, 214–217, 218–219
  laws, 64–65
  for stress, 132–133
Time, management of, 132
To Live Again (TLA), 183
Toilet training, 25
Transactional analysis, 131
Truman, Harry S., 117
Trust, need for, 222

Unconscious, collective, 107
Unemployment, in midlife,
  117–118

Viorst, Judith, 157
Vocational choices. *See* Career
  choices
Volunteerism, 177

Wants, universal, 219–222
*When All You Ever Wanted Isn't
  Enough* (Kushner), 212–213
Wills, for elderly, 201–202
Women. *See also* Menopause;
  Mothers
  creativity of, 182

Women (*cont.*)
  middle age adjustment, 108,
    109
  midlife career changes, 126–127
  sexual issues, 141
Work
  Freud on, 93
  in middle age, 112
  midlife stress and, 117–120
Work choices, *See* Career choices

Young adulthood
  age thirty transition, 94–95
  anxieties of, 68–69
  anxiety disorders in, 85–91
  career decisions, 73–74
  characteristics of, 67–68
  developmental tasks, 68–69,
    73–79
  emotional pressures of, 85–95
  leaving home, 69–71, 81
  life choices, 73–79
  love relationships, 74–76
  marriage in, 76–77
  parental appreciation in, 79–80
  parental guidelines for, 82–83
  parenthood in, 76–77
  responsibilities of, 68–69

ABOUT THE AUTHOR

H. MICHAEL ZAL, D.O., F.A.C.N., is a Board-Certified Psychiatrist who has maintained a private practice in Bala Cynwyd, Pennsylvania for the past twenty-one years. A graduate of the University of Pennsylvania and the Philadelphia College of Osteopathic Medicine, Dr. Zal completed a three-year National Institute of Mental Health Fellowship in Psychiatry through the Philadelphia Mental Health Clinic.

Dr. Zal is currently a clinical professor in the Department of Psychiatry at the Philadelphia College of Osteopathic Medicine. He is a Fellow of the American College of Neuropsychiatrists and a member of the University of Pennsylvania Private Practice Research Group. He is an attending physician at the Philadelphia Psychiatric Center and the Charter–Fairmount Institute, Philadelphia, Pennsylvania.

He is a lecturer on mental health topics as well as a medical writer and editor with numerous published articles to his credit. He was the winner of the 1988 Eric W. Martin Memorial Award, presented by the American Medical Writers Association, for outstanding writing. His winning article was "Panic Disorder—Is It Emotional Or Physical?", published in the July, 1987, issue of *Psychiatric Annals*. He is the author of *Panic Disorder: The Great Pretender,* published in 1990 by Plenum Press/ Insight Books.